HE'S JUST NOT UP FOR IT ANYMORE

why men stop

having sex,

and what you

can do about it

WILLIAM MORROW

An Imprint of HarperCollins*Publishers*

HE'S JUST NOT
UP FOR IT
ANYMORE

BOB BERKOWITZ, Ph.D., and
SUSAN YAGER-BERKOWITZ

HE'S JUST NOT UP FOR IT ANYMORE. Copyright © 2008 by Bob Berkowitz and Susan Yager-Berkowitz. All rights reserved. Printed in the United States of America. No part of this book may be used or reproduced in any manner whatsoever without written permission except in the case of brief quotations embodied in critical articles and reviews. For information address HarperCollins Publishers, 10 East 53rd Street, New York, NY 10022.

HarperCollins books may be purchased for educational, business, or sales promotional use. For information please write: Special Markets Department, HarperCollins Publishers, 10 East 53rd Street, New York, NY 10022.

FIRST EDITION

Designed by Susan Walsh

Library of Congress Cataloging-in-Publication Data has been applied for.

ISBN 978-0-06-119203-6

08 09 10 11 12 WBC/RRD 10 9 8 7 6 5 4 3 2 1

For Susan, the love of my life
B.B.

As always, for Bob
S.Y.B.

contents

HE'S JUST NOT

UP FOR IT

ANYMORE

INTRODUCTION

You know, it was hard on my ego and self-esteem when he didn't want me sexually, because I didn't grow up knowing there were men out there like that. **(Female, 40)**

It was strange to me how my interest in my wife died. I considered her an attractive woman, but she was always very angry. Her anger grew and grew until it became like she was actually seething whenever she looked at me. Even during all that time (twenty years) I was still attracted to her. But one day it was like a switch flipped off and I realized that I could no longer torture myself by being attracted to a woman who obviously hated me. **(Man, 50s)**

A woman we know once told us that although her marriage was otherwise wonderful, her husband of twelve years rarely had sex with her, and when he did, he appeared distant and detached. She felt positive he was faithful, straight, and not spending time with pornography. He just wasn't that interested, and she was confused. Was this the way she wanted to live for the rest of her life? So she went to a therapist. "What kind of woman have I become if I am willing to live this way?" she asked. "I'm very sexual, or at least I used to be. How can I have made this bargain? I have a good marriage except for one little thing—there's no sex. Don't I deserve more? Shouldn't I want more?" Her therapist replied that she was a sensible and mature woman, but much too hard on herself and her marriage. "Sex takes up such a small part of your life, at best 3 percent once you settle into a marriage. Why would you throw away something that's positive 97 percent of the time? Let's try to find out what's going on here."

The therapist helped our friend and her husband understand and improve their situation. Once they identified and accepted what was stopping the man from being passionate, desire was restored. Their issues, by the way, were not one-sided. They rarely are. Although on the surface they were best friends and thoroughly enjoyed each other's company, the couple had deeper problems, mainly his fear of intimacy and her tendency to be controlling and critical. The more he shut down emotionally, the more critical she became; the marriage and his libido were caught in a feedback loop. He was so afraid of being abandoned that he refused to allow real intimacy or commitment to enter his life, and the more she felt rejected, the more controlling and critical she became. But after addressing their problems, they say they are much happier and closer now in what they laughingly call their "second" marriage.

One thing they learned was not just to talk (they were already doing that) but to listen. Really listen, between the lines if necessary. Talking is a great first step, but listening is crucial; it allowed their marriage to adapt and then grow.

Unfortunately, other relationships aren't (or don't allow themselves to be) so blessed, and they deteriorate over the years. The following comment is from a woman whose husband seems to have shut down completely.

It's not just the fifteen years without ANY sex...it's the last three years of no touching, hugging, or kissing. My husband never says "I love you." He has killed my spirit. We have been married for thirty-three years and have four grown children. I am terrified to be alone at this point in my life, terrified of trying to support myself. But I am alone anyway, even if he is in the same room. I am now seriously thinking of divorce. I deserve better. **(Female, 50s)**

We agree with her. She does deserve better, and so does her spouse. They've lived together for what is likely more than half their lives. They've raised a family. But now they're alone, together. It's not difficult to understand her conflict. Her husband may be having similar doubts about their marriage now that the children are grown. What has made him reject her so completely? What happened fifteen years ago? Did he begin to suffer from erectile dysfunction, and chose abstinence or solitary sex over the possible humiliation of impotence? Was there a trauma she hasn't revealed? Did something make him so angry he's withholding sex as punishment? Does he suffer from depression? Is he on medication that is lowering his libido? There are many reasons why a man might stop being sexual with his partner, and often several of them overlap. She mentions that she is "terrified" of leaving the marriage, for economic as well as emotional reasons, and that is understandable.

"What kind of person have I become if I am willing to live without sex? Don't I deserve more?"

If food is scarce, it becomes important all the time; if readily available, it is just another part of life, and hopefully a delicious one.

When the sexual side of marriage is functioning well, it becomes a delectable but small portion of the total relationship. This 3 percent the therapist mentioned is only a tiny piece of your time, but just as small percentages of vitamins and minerals are necessary for a healthy diet, small portions of time together devoted to intimacy, tenderness, and passion are essential for a healthy marriage.

MAYBE IT'S COUNTERINTUITIVE, BUT IT'S OFTEN THE MAN'S DECISION

Living in a sexless marriage leaves you feeling isolated and lonely, especially when he's lying right there beside you every night. **(Female, 42)**

When we explained our project to a couple of our male friends, they were incredulous, which was interesting considering their professions. "Is that *really* a problem?" asked the gynecologist. Yes, we replied. It surely is. "Isn't it usually the *woman* who doesn't want to have sex?" the sociologist inquired. Absolutely not, we responded. Voluntary celibacy after you're married can be an equal gender opportunity.

It is now estimated that more than 20 million marriages in the United States are without physical passion. In other words, 15 to 20 percent of American couples have sex fewer than ten times per year. According to the United States Health and Social Life Survey (USHSL) of 1999, lack of desire is recognized as the most common sexual problem in America, affecting approximately 20 percent of the adult male, and 33 percent of the adult female population. However, since men are less likely to self-identify as being nonsexual, it is possible that the real number is even higher. Clinical psychologist David Schnarch, who runs the Family Health Center in Evergreen, Colorado, and has worked with couples and intimacy issues for over twenty years, states: "My clinical experience suggests more men struggle with low sexual desire than the study [USHSL, 1999] found. I'd guess sexual disinterest occurs equally frequently between men and women." Clinical psychologists Cathryn G. Pridal and Joseph LoPiccolo would agree. They believe that sociocultural shifts over the past two decades have resulted in women having a higher success rate in convincing their low-desire mates to seek help, and this is likely why no-sex marriages appear to be on the rise. In the 1990s, they wrote: "We recently studied our clinic's files and found that of all our low sexual desire cases, more than 70 percent of those seen in the 1970s were female, whereas of those seen thus far in the 1990s, the sex ratio was equally split between low drive males and low drive females. So although the total number of low desire cases is up, a good bit of this rise comes from the increase in male cases."

It is unusual for any two people to remain in complete sexual harmony after the initial phase of great and constant passion winds down. Most couples drift apart in their level of desire. They individualize a lot of other things, too, like the perfect time for dinner, what movie to see next, and how many televised sports events or antique stores are one too many. If the relationship is functioning well, they will compromise and reach satisfactory resolutions.

But we were curious about something other than how a low-libido and high-libido couple can find happiness; we wanted to know about men who were operating as if they had no libido at all. We wanted to research the underreported fact than many men are choosing to have little or no sex with their spouses, and try to understand why so many husbands are shutting down in this way. We also wanted to know how their wives were reacting and feeling and what they could do about it.

Human sexuality is a complex, delicate, and fragile thing. It can get derailed for as many reasons as there are sexually active people, and its absence can seriously damage and even end a relationship that might otherwise not only survive, but soar. For those who have been fortunate enough to find a partner whom they want to live with forever, a marriage suddenly devoid of intimacy can be puzzling, enraging, painful, and lonely.

> Due to the lack of sex, intimacy has stopped on all levels. We don't hold hands, hug, or even really talk anymore. It is so very isolating. Most of my women friends who are in sexless marriages are relieved, but I don't feel that way at all. I miss it very much. (Female, 45)

Since men often express emotions through sex, when they shut down emotionally, they often shut down sexually as well. It isn't possible to know why the man mentioned in the preceding quote has stopped being sexual, but it seems to have been going on for so long that he has detached himself on all levels. He no longer communicates about anything except trivia. As difficult as this is for his wife, it may be even more isolating for him. In our culture, men are often reluctant to reveal a lack of sexual desire, even to their closest friends. It equates with powerlessness and failure. Women, however, often do speak of such things, as the woman in the preceding quote is doing. It is interesting that she says most of her friends in sexless marriages are relieved, and they have no problem admitting neither they nor their husbands are sexually active.

> Thank you for doing this research. Just knowing there are other women who are going through what I have been going through for over thirty years is, in a strange way, comforting. (Female, 50s)

However, other women, like the one just quoted, are diffident about discussing intimate issues. They may fear embarrassment or want to avoid psychologically threatening conversation. They may consider it a betrayal of their partner, or just too personal to share with even their closest friends.

We surveyed men who stopped having sex with their wives and women whose husbands stopped having sex with them. More than 4,000 people responded.

We thoroughly enjoy the idea of marriage and feel unbelievably fortunate to be a part of one that is working well. However, when we say "marriage," "husband," or "wife," we are referring to any long-term committed relationship and the two people who make up that union. Besides, as we found out, a guy doesn't have to march down the aisle to stop making love to his partner. We also found out that although we are focusing on situations where men make the decision, a marriage without passion stems from multiple causes, frequently in combination, and rarely is only one person the catalyst. And although we are aware that homosexual relationships can also be without passion, we have restricted ourselves to heterosexual unions. It seems clear, however, that fear of intimacy, anger, boredom, depression, and low testosterone levels are relevant to all sexual orientations.

Our goal was to enlist a self-identified population of people in sexless marriages where the man was the one to initiate the end of intimacy. We surveyed men who stopped having sex with their wives and women whose husbands stopped having sex with them. Many respondents were generous enough to allow follow-up in-depth interviews; every participant was promised anonymity, and all responses were numerically coded to eliminate any possibility of identification. More than 4,000 people responded, 33 percent male and 67 percent female. A copy of the survey and significant data can be found in the appendix. In addition, we interviewed psychologists, sex therapists, and physicians—all leading experts in their fields—and thoroughly reviewed the literature, theories old and new, and relevant statistical data. Our approach was journalistic rather than scientific, and in all cases we tried to read and listen carefully, to really hear and respect what people were saying.

And talk they did, possibly welcoming an opportunity to discuss something that is not only painful, but, in contemporary Western society, an admission of failure. If you turn on the TV, go to the movies, or even open a magazine, everyone seems to be having a lot of sex. It can be incredibly difficult for a woman to think "He doesn't want me. I'm just not sexy to him anymore," or for a man to question his potency, skill, and, ultimately, masculinity. One 35-year-old woman said: "There are almost no resources for people in this situation." And a 30-year-old told us:

> The minute I became his wife he stopped seeing me as a sexual being. For example, he told me that wives should never wear sexy underwear. I am only 30 years old and feel a part of me has died. I believe in the marriage vows, but within a year of marriage I was thinking about divorce. I applaud you for writing this book. A man not wanting sex is a subject that is never discussed, and I hope women like me can be comforted by your research.

Men choosing not to be sexual with their wives is underreported and rarely talked about. Their wives are perplexed, and sometimes angry. One thing seems very clear. The women want answers, and they don't seem to be getting them from their silent partners.

PART I

the sexless husband

one

WHY MEN STOP HAVING SEX

Most women are raised to believe men want sex all the time, a belief the media consistently reinforces. So when a woman suddenly finds herself in a sexless marriage, it not only hurts a lot, it's bewildering. It seems irrational. That same man, the one who couldn't wait to get you alone, couldn't wait to make love to you, now acts either annoyed or exhausted if you even hint at intimacy. Sex should be such a natural, pleasurable, loving, simple thing, shouldn't it? How did this happen?

Sex, of course, isn't simple at all. It may be an expression of love, a whole lot of fun, irresistibly sublime, and the high point of your day, but simple it's not. Some anthropologists suggest it was, once upon a time. When the objective was procreation and a male perhaps shared meat with a female in exchange for as much sex as he wanted, both were far too busy hunting, gathering, and outrunning whatever creature might hunt and gather them first to worry about whether or not sex was happening on a regular basis. And, after all, who knew what a regular basis was, anyway?

Today we know, or at least we think we do. Women's magazines seem to constantly be giving results to polls that ask the inevitable question: "If you are married or in a committed relationship, how often do you have sex?" The average is one to two times a week, a figure that hasn't changed since Kinsey first published his data on men in 1948 and women in 1953. Data are data, but what about all the couples who wouldn't score quite so high on this test? If you are in a relationship where once a month is the norm, or for that matter, once a year, do you even want to take the test?

Why is it that so many married couples find themselves living a life of celibacy?

Today we live in a world where every available form of media seems to scream out that people, and men in particular, want sex, and more sex. That trite and hackneyed expression "sex sells" still seems to be the mantra for pushing everything from soda to cars, to, well, sex. And the majority of us buy into this. We want to be those elusive things—desirable and sexy. The ultimate goal, what most of us really want, or think we really want, is to fall so much in love, to be in a relationship so committed that we become one special person's own private sex symbol. We get a house together, and maybe a family, and lots of sex. Forever.

So why is it that so many married couples, those very people able to have as much sex as they want, find themselves living a life of celibacy? These same couples probably once had sex on a regular basis. They thought each other interesting, attractive, and desirable enough to commit to sharing a bed forever. What stopped the passion?

IF YOU'RE IN A SEXLESS MARRIAGE, YOU'RE NOT ALONE

It's good to know there are other women who experience this. I thought it was really rare. (Female, 35)

Surveys tell us that 40 million Americans live in a no-sex or low-sex marriage. Some believe the number might be even higher. After all, we live in a culture where everyone, or at least everyone in a committed relationship, is supposed to be having sex, and lots of it. Not having sex equals failure, a lack of desirability. Who wants to check the "never" box on that magazine quiz?

A sexless marriage is defined by experts as making love ten times a year or less. Whether or not that is a problem, of course, depends on the couple. If both are content, if "ten times a year or less" meets their needs and expectations, then they have no problem. Unfortunately, this usually is not the case. Often the loss of sexual pleasure and intimacy results in depression, suspicion, anger, resentment, and sometimes, infidelity and divorce. Although it is clear that this issue is rarely one-sided, it is nevertheless surprising to many that it is just as often the man who puts the brakes on sexuality as the woman. The late Dr. Bernie Zilbergeld, who was one of America's leading sex therapists, suggested it was *more* often the man when he wrote, " . . . in the vast amount of couples consulting me about desire complaints it's the women who want more and the man who always has a headache." These same men who used to do whatever it took to get their fiancées or new brides into bed no longer desire them. What happened?

WHAT STOPS THE PASSION?

Why *do* men stop having sex with their wives? The reason is seldom simple and may have a physiological, psychological, or cultural foundation; recent studies add a genetic component. Often these elements combine.

We looked at the statistical reasons our male survey respondents, who self-identified as choosing not to have sex with their spouses, gave us for no longer being intimate, and we studied their comments carefully. Let's first take a look at some statistics. We asked men to rate a list of reasons on a scale that went from strongly agree to strongly disagree. The following table lists in descending order the percentage of men who agreed with each of the causes.

WHY MEN SAID THEY STOPPED

REASON	PERCENTAGE (%)
She isn't sexually adventurous enough for me.	68
She doesn't seem to enjoy sex.	61
I am interested in sex with others, but not with my wife.	48
I am angry at her.	44
I'm bored.	41
She is depressed.	40
She has gained a significant amount of weight.	38
I am depressed.	34
I no longer find her physically attractive.	32
I suffer from erectile dysfunction.	30
I lost interest and I don't know why.	28
I prefer to masturbate, but not online.	25*
I prefer to watch pornography online and masturbate.	25*
I am on medication that lowered my libido.	21
I am/was having an affair.	20
I suffer from premature ejaculation.	16
I have difficulty achieving orgasm.	15
I am too tired.	14
She is/was having an affair.	9
I don't have the time.	6
I wasn't interested in sex to begin with.	3
I am gay.	<1

*These figures may overlap.

Even an anonymous online survey might cause some people to reshape or shade the truth. Although the men know (or at least *think* they know) the reasons for their voluntary celibacy but the women are only guessing, either way the situation is embarrassing and painful. It is therefore not surprising that both men and women agree most with statements that shift responsibility away from themselves. Indeed, men indicate a lack of sexual adventure (hers, not his) as primary. It is difficult to believe that this lack of erotic excitement is completely one-sided, and that these men who identify their wives as unadventurous are themselves imaginatively passionate guys, just somehow mysteriously unable to inspire the one woman they chose to marry.

Both men and women agree most with statements that shift responsibility away from themselves.

After all, they probably knew her acceptable level of tolerance for erotic exploration before the vows were exchanged. We suspect that boredom or other factors is closer to the truth, or they are confusing the pornography they see on DVDs or the Internet with reality.

STOP THE PRESSES! THESE MEN REALLY *DO* WANT SEX!

The overwhelming majority of men who responded to our survey seem to indicate that they are still sexually active beings, or would like to be. The few exceptions are those with seriously debilitating medical conditions, and the 3 percent who said they never wanted sex to begin with. Slightly less than half say they are interested in sex, but not with their partners, which might be valid but could also mean boredom, anger, or performance anxiety. The majority masturbates, online or off, indicating a possible predilection for solitary over partnered sex. And although only 25 percent indicated a preference for masturbating to online porn, 58 percent said yes, they looked at it. For many of these men, a fantasy world is replacing an actual sex life with their spouse, bringing to mind the Oscar Wilde quote: "One's real life is often the life one does not lead."

THEN WHY AREN'T THEY MAKING LOVE TO THEIR WIVES?

Here are some of the main reasons we believe men in partnered relationships choose celibacy or solitary sex. The issues are rarely one-sided or stand alone; indeed, they often combine. This is an overview, and all will be discussed in greater depth later on in the book. It should be mentioned here that the following list is by no means complete, it just represents the majority. A few men appear to come from backgrounds so traumatic (e.g., sexual, physical, or emotional abuse) that a fear of intimacy or dependency makes sustaining an intimate partnered relationship impossible without extensive psychological counseling. Others are alcohol or drug dependent to a degree that disallows a satisfactory sexual relationship, and still others suffer from physical illness and disease that precludes sex.

He's Bored/She's Bored

Drs. Max and Della Fitzgerald are clinical sex therapists who studied with William Masters and Virginia Johnson and are founders of The Fitzgerald Institute in North Carolina. We asked them why they believed some men stop having sex with their wives. Max replied that the main reason is boredom. "Same place, same station. We do it the same way every time. Men like variety, and when a couple gets stuck in a routine, the man is the first one to get dissatisfied with it." Della agreed, saying, "Definitely, boredom."

Doing the same thing over and over again and expecting different results is that wonderful definition of insanity attributed to Albert Einstein. It often is what happens in the conjugal bed. What seemed exciting once upon a time now seems just plain dull. Some men may not be having sex with their wives because sex simply isn't worth the effort. They'd rather watch television. Their wives may feel the same way, not really missing mediocre sex, just missing that feeling of being desired.

Why does sex become predictable and boring?

This lack of newness, energy, and emotion translates for many men into a lack of adventure and sexual enjoyment on the part of their partners, transferring the problem and ignoring the fact that they're not bringing any originality to bed, either. What they are really feeling here is rejection, thinking, "My spouse lacks enthusiasm for, and is apathetic about—*me*! She doesn't care about *me* anymore. If she did, she would be more passionate!"

Why does married sex become predictable and boring? Dr. Helen Fisher, a research professor of anthropology at Rutgers University, divides love into three categories—lust, romantic love, and attachment—and considers these to be evolved drives associated with different brain chemicals. Lust inspires us to seek a range of partners. Romantic love drives us, instead, to focus on a specific romantic partner. We often fall romantically in love with someone we perceive, perhaps subconsciously, to be a good provider and to father the type of children we want (if we are female), and likely to conceive and nurture the type of children we want (if we are male). In those exhilarating early days of romance, our beloved seems fascinating, irresistible, and red hot. These are the glory days long-term married couples wistfully remember—the "honeymoon" stage (that sometimes doesn't even last until the honeymoon) when desire for each other was a constant, rather than a sometime, thing. Most couples made love every day, some multiple times a day; at any rate, when two people fall into lust that leads to love, the brain chemicals necessary to best ensure propagation of the species are distributed in just the right amounts to make them want to make love all the time. However, Dr. Fisher believes that "it is not adaptive to be intensely romantically in love for twenty years. . . . [And] we would all die of sexual exhaustion." In a good relationship, brain chemicals shift and attachment emerges. This is the sense of calm and peace, a Sunday kind of love that is the foundation of a stable, long-term partnership, enabling the pair to raise their offspring. It trumps lust, at least most of the time. Ironically, hormones that allow attachment to thrive (oxytocin and vasopressin) suppress lust and romantic love. It would appear to be a catch-22—great marriage, or great sex.

Clinical psychologist and sex therapist David Schnarch agrees that marriage, and the readily available sex that goes along with it, frequently results in partners wanting less instead of more. Schnarch makes a psychological rather than biological case for decreased passion, arguing that "the person with the least desire for sex always controls the frequency of sexual contact between spouses." Thus, if a man stops wanting sex because of fear (erectile dysfunction [ED], premature ejaculation, inhibited orgasm, fathering a child, intimacy issues), anger, or depression, and his wife becomes accustomed to and distressed by what she experiences as his rejection of herself, she will ultimately stop trying to reverse the trend. The converse is true as well. The wife may be refusing the husband for her own reasons, until he no longer feels the effort is worthwhile. They might even be on a sexual seesaw, each taking turns being the one pursuing or turning away.

Dr. Schnarch believes that there is a clear correlation between the increasing importance of one's partner to oneself and the unsettling discomfort of being vulnerable. The fear of losing a spouse, or having a spouse choose to leave, can result in decreased desire as a protective mechanism. The more complete the relationship, the greater the loss if it ends. That's why, he suggests, some people find it easier to experiment in one-night stands or emotionally disposable affairs—there's no risk of being exposed, rejected, or considered deviant when the other person can't hurt you. Schnarch states: "We demand stability in marriage—and when we get it we complain things are always the same."

Familiarity Breeds Contentment

These are intriguing theories, but can anything be done to alleviate the boredom? There are no easy solutions to the monotonous sex that evolves in many marriages, but if the problem is just fatigue with the sex-by-numbers, don't-do-anything-surprising or don't-take-any-chances routine that married sex often becomes, then *anything* different usually works. (That's why so many couples have sex the minute they get to their vacation hotel room, jet lag or no jet lag. It's not the free time or the lack of day-to-day pressure; it's the change of venue, the different bed, sheets, and pajamas that liberate.) All those magazine solutions—lingerie, massages, erotica, fantasies, and sex toys—can help, for a short time, at least. There's a lot to be said for a silk camisole and high heels instead of a torn T-shirt and socks. The problem is, eventually you run out of ideas and money. Dr. Schnarch (and others) makes a strong case for differentiation, which is holding on to your own identity and looking to *yourself* for approval and validation, and not your spouse. We concur.

The constant, relentless, delicious sex of those first few months or years will probably never return.

Individuality and separateness encourages passion and is probably imperative in retaining heat in your marriage, or restarting the fire.

But we want to make an important point here: The constant, relentless, delicious sex of those first few months or years will probably never return.

For the majority of people fortunate enough to be in loving long-term committed relationships, fantasies, vacations, and lacy underwear aren't going to reverse those brain chemicals back to the good old days, or exorcise every last one of those vulnerability demons. They might jump-start things a bit, and probably will, as long as both partners are open to change, and there are no other issues to deal with, which is often not the case. And even in the most optimal of relationships there are, apart from the workday itself, the mundane routines necessary to keep the household going—bills to be paid, groceries shopped for, meals prepared and dishes washed, garbage taken out, not to mention the kids. Even if these chores are shared reasonably, married life is still very different from those early months of dating. The everyday aspects of a well-functioning marriage are not to be trivialized; they can in fact be calming and build contentment and security, but sexy they're not. And all the magazine articles in the world telling you to light a bunch of candles and run an aromatic bath can't explain *how* to transition from a steamy hot soak to a steamy hot night of sex.

Sexual Novocain

Anger is a powerful sexual Novocain, and 44 percent of the men said they were furious. They felt criticized and controlled, undervalued and insignificant, yet many couldn't, or wouldn't, talk about it with their partners. Afraid of yet another fight, or a long list of things they're doing wrong, they shut down emotionally and sexually.

> My wife is so overly critical, in every possible way, starting with my work, telling me what I should or shouldn't be doing and telling me how I should be living my life. She treats me like a child, saying things like "If you don't put your shoes away, I'm going to throw them outside the door." (Male, 47)

Clearly, the marriage described in the preceding quote is filled with bitterness and disappointment. The wife has become an annoying bully; he has shut down completely and withholds the only thing he thinks might hurt her. They probably both feel underappreciated.

Couples need to learn how to discuss their issues with respect, and to really listen to each other.

We have to wonder what benefit each is getting from this seemingly unhappy partnership. Do they find comfort in their assigned roles of nagging wife and henpecked husband, reenacting unpleasant yet familiar scenes from their childhood? Does the wife's constant criticism give her husband the needed psychological ammunition to withdraw from her sexually? Is that something he would want to do anyway?

> I'm angry at her because she knows it all and always has to be right. She wants to keep talking about things until I'm sick of it. (Male, 49)

This comment interested us because it seemed to indicate an unfortunate but common marital problem. She keeps talking, but he stopped listening. He may feel like the junior partner and since she "always has to be right," he believes there is no room for his opinion or feelings. At this point, negative communication appeals to her more than none at all. The problem is there's no real conversation going on here. Her plan is to keep speaking until she gets him to agree with her—she's desperate for his understanding and support—and this is unlikely because, to him, it's all nagging and he tuned out long ago. His plan is to communicate silently, by withholding sex. Couples need to learn how to discuss their issues with respect, and to really listen to each other. She has to begin by trying to explain what's re*ally* bothering her, and he has to try to slow down, stop, and hear what she's saying.

I'm just plain mad. I do so much more around the house than my father ever did: I vacuum, wash dishes, do the laundry, and change the diapers. I want what women have been saying they want for years, thanks and respect. I want to feel wanted. And until I get it, there isn't going to be any sex. (Male, 50s)

We strongly believe egalitarian marriages work best, and we also think partners *should* thank each other for doing those little, usually unpleasant, boring, and, yes, thankless, jobs. This guy feels not only unappreciated, but unwanted. Sadly, he has become a twenty-first-century-male Lysistrata, withholding sex until his personal battle for respect is won.

For my own amusement, I took to counting the seconds between arriving home from work every day and the first negative comment. It was generally significantly less than a minute. (Male, 50s)

Most men tie their self-worth into two things: their sexuality and their jobs. Unfortunately for them, this is the very foundation of their validation, and it easily gets cracked and eroded. If a woman shows a man no passion (in spite of the fact that he may not have any himself), he will feel rejected, and the rejection will, often, turn into anger, apathy, or depression. A little bit of flattery might go a long way in the situation described in the previous quote, but any kind of positive reinforcement tends to be one of the first things to exit from an anger-based marriage. What remains is an emotional void, a relationship where intimacy becomes foreign and distasteful, and not to be trusted because the risk is far greater than the reward.

An angry man may be a raging bull, or he may just sit quietly, secretly consumed by fury.

No Erection = No Sex

Forty percent of men over the age of 40 suffer from impotence at least on occasion, and the percentage increases with age. It is estimated that more than 30 million men in the United States have this problem. Certain medical conditions, such as hypertension, diabetes, and obesity, can result in difficulty getting or maintaining an erection. Depression and anxiety can have the same result, as can many and various medications (including some used for treating depression and anxiety). Losing the ability to get and maintain an erection goes to the very core of masculinity, and it can be easier to just stop having (partnered) sex than risk embarrassment. And, by the way, only a small percentage of men who could benefit from Viagra, Cialis, or Levitra get prescriptions. Impotence is that difficult to discuss, even with a doctor. It seems probable that it is underreported even in an anonymous online survey.

Although 30 percent of the male respondents acknowledged problems with ED, 39 percent of the women thought it was a problem. The men who were willing to admit it was an issue rarely commented further, and when they did it was often to transfer the source of their "problem" to the woman they married, suggesting that her lack of adventure, interest, or even her appearance was the real reason.

Later in the book we will explain the physiological and psychological reasons for erectile dysfunction, as well as the closely related problems of premature ejaculation and inhibited orgasm, and explore ways to approach and solve this problem with compassion and tact and help you or your partner stop suffering in silence. It is an extremely common problem, and, importantly, one that usually can be easily resolved.

Depression and Libido-Lowering Medications

Clinical sex therapist Della Fitzgerald believes depression is one of the main reasons men stop being sexual with their wives, and the majority of our female respondents agree. Dr. Fitzgerald states: "Many times the man may not even be aware that he is depressed over the stressful things in life—economic stress, career stress, not achieving the things he wants. He is not even aware he has responded [to the stress] with anger, and the anger has gone underground and moved into depression. He is not enthusiastic about anything at all." He is not enthusiastic about having sex with his wife if he thinks *she's* depressed, either. That was the case with almost four out of ten men.

Ironically, just as depression lowers libido, so do many antidepressants. There are new ones on the market now that are supposed to have less of a libido-lowering effect; however, everyone reacts individually to these drugs, or combination of drugs. It is imperative they be prescribed by a specialist such as a psychiatrist or psychopharmacologist. Often, if a drug reduces sexual desire, it can be switched with one that won't. It is extremely important that you inquire about any negative side effects that may occur, and discuss them fully with the physician, pharmacist, and your spouse.

SSRI = So Sorry, Romance Impossible?

Dr. Helen Fisher believes that some of these drugs (selective serotonin reuptake inhibitors, or SSRIs, such as, for example, Zoloft and Prozac) may not only lower libido, but also prevent the development of romantic love and attachment. They may even eliminate the ability to have those feelings, making a person in a committed long-term relationship suddenly and inexplicably feel no longer in love with his or her partner.

We are in no way suggesting that a depressed person should not get help (nor did anyone we interviewed); we think that these medications can make life worth living again and even save lives. However, we do believe antidepressants are sometimes prescribed for specious reasons, or without full disclosure, or, as an absolute worst-case scenario, just borrowed from a friend, and used without any medical supervision at all. Depression, like impotence, can be a sign of masculinity gone astray, and difficult to admit, even to oneself.

Virtual Sex

Men have used various forms of erotica for partnered enhancement and solitary pleasure for centuries. Erotic artifacts, some dating back thousands of years, have been found in archaeological digs. However, until very recently, pornography was limited to printed material (which allowed for rich fantasies) and seedy movie houses. The VCR made privacy possible, but content was limited and not readily accessible. The Internet irrevocably changed all that. Now every type of exotic erotica is available, and it's private, cheap, and virtually infinite. This is the biggest, newest, and most versatile sex toy of them all.

Why would a guy spend so much time online looking at naked women when he has one in bed, ready, willing, and able?

Some men view porn as a way to have imaginary sex with other women without actually cheating on their wives. There are also examples of chat rooms leading to virtual adultery and online infidelity; whether these are crimes or misdemeanors can only be determined by the couple involved. Others use the stimulation to enhance their offline experiences, and sometimes ask their partners to join in. And clearly, some guys are using porn as a complete substitute for marital sex, like this 45-year-old male who wrote:

> When I was a kid, I used to love *Penthouse* and *Playboy*. What guy didn't? But the Internet has opened up this whole world of endless pornographic experiences, beyond my wildest dreams.

I feel guilty, but after the first few years of marriage, my wife just can't compete. I still love her, but I have no desire to have sex with her anymore.

If a woman is married to a man like this, it's bewildering:

I really can't figure out why it happened. I was willing to have sex with him at any given time, but he just kept watching [porn] more and more. He would tell me it was going to stop. He would hide it from me and I would catch him. I keep getting angrier and more resentful. We are on a downward spiral, and the madder I get, the more he rejects me and watches porn. I think he enjoys it more than he enjoys it with real women, certainly more than with this real woman. **(Female, 40s)**

Why would a guy spend so much time online looking at naked women when he has one in bed, ready, willing, and able? Well, there's the variety, of course, and he knows for sure that he'll get lucky. There's no pressure of any kind, no performance anxiety, no emotion, no talk, no criticism, no foreplay. Anyone else's pleasure is irrelevant. He's insulated from rejection and perceived inadequacies. It may be light-years away from connected, committed, hot (or spiritual) sex, but it's quick, it's easy, and it doesn't require an erection. (Male sexual pleasure and ejaculation are most definitely possible without one.) If getting or maintaining an erection is problematical, online porn can be a refuge.

He's into You, He's Just Not That into Sex

Inhibited sexual desire (ISD, also termed "asexual") affects about 1 percent of the population. It is a rare condition where desire is, and always has been, completely absent. Hypoactive sexual desire disorder (HSDD) is more widespread and is defined by the American Psychiatric Association as any "deficiency" or "absence of sexual fantasies and desire for sexual activity," producing "personal or interpersonal distress," that is not a result of a psychological illness such as depression, a medical condition, or libido-lowering medications, alcohol, or drug abuse. This definition is intentionally broad, omitting qualifiers such as age, physical condition, and whether or not there is any "normal" level of desire, suggesting that "normal" would be whatever is necessary not to produce distress. In many cases of HSDD, appetite for physical intimacy is low, but once aroused, satisfactory performance and pleasure follow. In other words, a significant number of guys do want sex, just not a lot of it.

She Gained a Lot of Weight

There is no getting around the fact that 32 percent of our male respondents claimed they stopped having sex with their wives because they no longer found them attractive, and 38 percent said the reason was weight gain. Clearly, these may be cover-ups for depression, anger, or impotence. It is always easier to obfuscate blame, especially when the problem is, at least in part, yourself. So, let us make this clear before we write another sentence—we aren't talking about a few extra pounds, which, without question, are an excuse, not a reason. However, if a woman is more than around thirty pounds overweight, her partner may be telling the truth. Men are visual, perhaps even more so than women, so excessive weight gain may indeed be a problem for them. Mysteriously, whether or not they themselves have added extra pounds, too, is irrelevant.

More Weight, Less Want

Obesity also diminishes libido, so an overweight person may not be as responsive a partner as he or she once was. There is also new evidence that correlates male obesity and impotence. Mix obesity, ED, and low libido together and it may be easier to just stop trying. (Conversely, a few men said the problem was that their wives *lost* weight.) Interestingly, *only one guy mentioned that he would prefer a younger woman.*

With obesity at an all-time high in America, it is not a surprise that weight gain is an issue. Some men might interpret it as just one more rejection—another example that she no longer loves and respects him. If he looks a bit deeper, of course, he'll realize that she no longer respects herself, either.

He's Not Too Tired, and He's Got the Time

A *Newsweek* cover (June 30, 2003) photographs an attractive heterosexual couple in bed. She's visibly confused and distressed, soothing her pain by spooning chocolate Häagen-Dazs straight from the carton; her guy is intently at work on his laptop, barely aware of her presence. She might as well be alone, as suggested by the headline "No Sex Please, We're Married—Are Stress, Kids and Work Killing Romance?" Women's magazines often reinforce this theory of DINS (dual income, no sex) couples. They say that for many of us, long hours at work, child care, and other responsibilities leave little time or energy left over for lovemaking. We are stressed out, or just plain exhausted, and have forgotten how to make time for love. This seems like a convincing argument, and often goes on to suggest ways to fit your spouse back into your life, culminating, usually, with the inevitable idea of "date nights"; in other words, penciling romance into your schedule and trying hard not to cross it off for something more appealing—as if sex were just one more tedious chore to check off your "to do" list.

Forcing sex back into your life won't work. However, it is important to make time for each other, and not forget why you fell in love in the first place; indeed, to remember when you could always find time to be with your partner, because when you first met that was a top priority. A walk in the park, a movie, dinner out, and *any* time alone, especially away from the kids, is critical. It will bring you closer, it will be different, and no matter what happens, you both win.

Now, is he too tired or not? Although 44 percent of our female respondents thought that their husbands *were* too tired to be intimate, a mere 14 percent of the men agreed with this. Neither women (18%) nor men (6%) bought into the worn-out excuse of not enough time, perhaps remembering that if you want to do something badly enough, you can always figure out a way to pencil it in.

Why do women think guys are tired when they aren't? Well, it can be another shift of responsibility, a belief that if *he* wasn't tired, everything would be fine. Or the men's fatigue might be an indicator of depression, something, as we mentioned earlier, guys are often reluctant to admit. It can also be a convenient cover-up for impotence, anger, boredom, or the unfortunate fact that he masturbated to online porn right before going to bed.

He's Having an Affair

Has this happened because he is having an affair, or is he just not in love with me? How do you know when your husband will not talk to you about it? (Woman, 40s)

Another woman? Not likely. Only 20 percent of the men said they had, or were currently having, an affair. This number is slightly lower than the one published by the University of Chicago's National Opinion Research Center (21.2%), or the 2006 Elle Magazine/MSNBC survey dealing with long-term relationships and sex in America (21%).

Curiously, most men who *were* unfaithful did not seem to indicate any desire to leave their wives. This man (61) has been married to his wife (56) for thirty years:

I have had many affairs with other women. One of those is long-term. Yes, I've replaced my wife's role as my sex partner, but I haven't replaced her emotionally.

He indicates that he loves his wife, and wants to share his life with no one else, but is no longer aroused by her. While it's possible that he needs new partners, and/or the excitement of cheating to perform, it's equally possible that a fear of intimacy is preventing him from committing fully to the woman he loves. He doesn't say if his wife has a sexual surrogate of her own, but we strongly doubt he thinks she does.

And this man has been married for sixteen years:

> I was faithful for the first fifteen years of our marriage, even though she stopped being intimate—emotionally, not sexually— with me after five or six years. About a year ago I started having an affair with a woman I met on a business trip. I really like her, but I'm so afraid if I remarry the whole thing will happen all over again. Also, I don't want to leave my 13-year-old son. (Male, 46)

The man in the preceding quote is interesting for a variety of reasons. He breaks the stereotype that men want sex and women want love; he is openly admitting that he wants more of an emotional connection than he believes his wife is capable of giving. However, he doesn't seem to have discussed this with her, or explored why their fifteen-year marriage has been, at least to him, emotionally starved for the last nine or ten years. What happened after year five? Instead of looking for causatives, he's using the problem as an excuse for an affair—shifting responsibility for his behavior from himself to his wife. And now he wants it all—wife, son, and mistress.

Of course, this guy will likely have to leave his captain's paradise, one way or the other. His empty promises may transform the mistress into a less available woman, giving him a convenient reason to reject her, too. Or she may just get tired of his false promises and leave. His wife may discover his secret, and, if so, he stands a good chance of losing his son's respect along with his marriage.

It is theorized that many if not most couples do not survive the revelation of an affair, even if it is dealt with in couple's therapy, probably because it is the most often cited reason for divorce. However, it seems clear that honest and controlled statistics are difficult to obtain, and that the couples who choose not to divorce but work through their painful issues privately cannot be quantified. It is possible, perhaps, with counseling and definitely with hard work, to use the pain of infidelity as a catalyst for change, that is, as a way of finding out what is preventing a real relationship.

The vast majority of men, even if they aren't making love to their wives, aren't making love to anyone else, either.

At the end of our survey, the question was phrased differently. We asked "Did you have an affair *after* [italics ours] you stopped having sex with your wife?" and the percentage increased to 27 percent. Those men seemed to be longing for validation—someone to say that they were lovable, acceptable, and, above all, desirable.

> I had forgotten what it was like to have a woman actually desire me and want to be with me physically. We talked on the phone daily for at least two hours. When we had our weekly trysts, we would spend as much time talking as making love. **(Man, 50)**

Of course, there are men who can't be validated enough no matter what their wife, lover, girlfriend, virtual pen pal, or anyone else tells them. There simply isn't enough love in the world to make them feel worthwhile. They need therapy to exist within a committed relationship. The thing to focus on is this: The vast majority of men, even if they aren't making love to their wives, aren't making love to anyone else, either. They may say their wives lack adventure, but they aren't, for the most part, looking elsewhere to find it.

He's Gay . . . or Is He?

Is our marriage just a cover for homosexuality? (Female, 59)

Sometimes a woman in a sexless marriage thinks that maybe, just maybe, her husband is gay. It would explain a lot, and take the responsibility off her completely. There would be no "other woman" to contend with. Divorce might be inevitable, but guilt free. In our survey, some women even expressed hope that this was the case.

About 4 percent of the male population is homosexual; this percentage goes up to an average of 9 percent in the twelve-largest American cities. Of course, the vast majority of gay men choose same-sex partners, making it possible, but highly improbable, that your husband is gay. So, we'll say it again. He probably has no other sex partner than his imagination.

two

WHY WOMEN THINK THEIR HUSBANDS STOP HAVING SEX

I've tried all sorts of things to interest him—suggestive comments, coming to bed naked, lingerie. So far nothing has worked and I'm really at a loss. **(Female, 30)**

Many women seem to be reaching into their sexual bag of tricks but, sadly, what once resulted in passionate sex is now met with indifference. It is extremely confusing to have the man you planned on sharing your life, dreams, *everything* with suddenly reject you. It hurts; and to compound the problem, most men don't want to talk about it, leaving their wives to try and solve the mystery without any clues.

We asked our female survey respondents (none of whom are married to the male respondents) why they believed their husbands stopped being sexual with them. These women had all self-identified as being in sexless marriages where the decision to stop being sexual was determined by their partners. As we did with the men, we asked women to rate a list of possible contributory factors on a scale that went from strongly agree to strongly disagree. The following table lists in descending order the percentage of women who agreed with each of the causes.

WHY WOMEN THINK THEIR PARTNERS STOPPED

REASON	PERCENTAGE (%)
He lost interest and I don't know why.	66
He is depressed.	57
He is angry at me.	45
He is too tired.	44
He no longer finds me physically attractive.	40
He suffers from erectile dysfunction.	39
I am depressed.	36
He's bored.	31
I have gained a significant amount of weight.	28
He has difficulty achieving orgasm.	27
He prefers to masturbate, but not while online.	27*
He prefers to watch pornography online and masturbate.	27*
He is on medication that lowered his libido.	26
He is interested in sex with other people, but not me.	25
He suffers from premature ejaculation.	20
He is/was having an affair.	19
He wasn't interested in sex to begin with.	19
He doesn't have the time.	18
I am not sexually adventurous enough.	14
I don't seem to enjoy sex.	10
I am/was having an affair.	9
He is gay.	2

*These figures may overlap.

A sexless marriage is so degrading to the woman, and it takes away her self-esteem. It's a lonely married life. **(Female, 58, married forty years)**

To be abandoned as a sexual partner by someone you have loved and trusted can corrode confidence and destroy once strong feelings of sensuality and femininity. It is not surprising that so many women (66%) said they didn't know why this happened, indicating that they were bewildered, confused, and just making an educated guess. Like the men, responsibility shifts away from themselves. Their partners are described as depressed and angry; they, for the most part, are adventurous and enjoy sex.

At times our female respondents describe extraordinary situations—for example, partners who appear to come from backgrounds so traumatic (sexual, physical, or emotional abuse) that a fear of dependency makes sustaining an intimate relationship impossible without extensive psychological counseling. These men often destroy any chance of closeness with multiple infidelities and/or complete indifference to their partners.

> My husband was sexually molested by his father, and, in my opinion he has not learned how to overcome this experience. I am not sure whether he is gay or not interested in sex. I honestly don't know. All I know is that I want it and need it. I'm 34 and men hit on me all the time. One day, who knows?

Other men are depicted as alcohol or drug dependent to a degree that disallows a satisfactory sexual relationship; or, sadly, others suffer from physical illness that irrevocably precludes or limits sexuality.

> My husband has several health issues, including type 2 diabetes. Perhaps because of that I should not have responded to the survey. However, while the health issues are the primary cause of our sexless marriage, the fact that he has done little to improve his health is a significant factor. I do, to some extent, perceive that as his "choosing" a sexless existence. (Female, 30s)

This woman typifies many who complained that their husbands had a condition that interfered with their performing adequately, but refused to either alter their lifestyle or seek medical help. It is possible that these men are using their medical problems as an excuse to stop being sexual with their wives, and are comfortable with the way things are.

When it comes to sexual equipment, almost all men fall well into the satisfactorily serviceable range, but that doesn't mean they believe it. However, only two women suggested that their husband's insecurity about penis size might be a contributing factor, although they may also be laughing at the enemy:

> He doesn't think he can satisfy me. He is very self-conscious about his size. (Female, 27)

> He also has a very small penis. (Female, 52)

It has been theorized that size once mattered a lot. The human male has a large penis compared with other, comparable, mammals. For example, a 160-pound man has an average erection of five and a half inches, a 400-pound gorilla averages one inch. Size may have been an indication of power and strength to primitive females. A large penis may have been used to impress and intimidate other males, and thus eliminate them as sexual rivals. Either way, the well-endowed male had a better chance of mating with young and fertile partners, and just possibly, the larger size got his sperm closer to the cervix so he had a better chance of impregnating them as well.

Although it has been conventional wisdom for decades that size doesn't count, to a lot of men (and some women), it does. Our Google search for "penile enhancement" got 1,480,000 results, countless advertisements, and spam we never even dreamed existed.

It is highly unlikely, however, that size would cause a man to stop being sexual with a longtime partner, unless, in anger, she made a cruel, nonretractable comment.

A man has a hard time admitting that he never cared about sex; so much of his personal net worth is tied into his sexuality.

And then there were the women who thought that sex was not on their guy's agendas right from the start. Nineteen percent agreed that "he was never that into sex to begin with." Men overwhelmingly disagreed, only 3 percent said this was a possibility. A man has a hard time admitting that he never cared about sex; so much of his personal net worth is tied into his sexuality.

> Before we were married I was not getting as much sex as I wanted. He would tell me that I was being unreasonable and he just didn't want it as much as I did. **(Female, 32)**

He's Depressed

American physicians wrote 118 million prescriptions for antidepressants in 2005, so it is not surprising that so many women believe their nonsexual spouses are depressed. It has been estimated that half of all couples seeking therapy for marital issues have at least one clinically depressed partner, and often, the more obviously symptomatic masks depression in the other. If, indeed, only one is depressed, the other may exacerbate the situation by trying to get his/her partner to "snap out of it." It is indisputable that depression causes a loss of libido, and so do some, but not all, medications to alleviate it.

> I think that he may not ever have been very interested in sex. The signs were there before we got married, but I ignored them. Halfway through our marriage, I think depression kicked

in so he wasn't able to fake it and even try anymore. He never initiated and turned me down at least half the time I initiated. (Female, 40)

Interestingly, 57 percent of the women said they believed their husbands were depressed, but only 34 percent of the men agreed they were. However, 40 percent of the male respondents thought their wives depressed.

He's Very Angry at Me

Almost half of all respondents agree—these men are angry! Some women can't explain it at all: "I'm not sure why he is angry at me. I just know that he is." Some think they can: "He has never succeeded in business, and actually came to work with me in the business that I own. I realize this could be emasculating for him. I try to let him know I value him for the work he does, but he still insults me constantly."

Anger at the trivial can mask anger at things too painful to explore.

Many women admit to being critical, aware that this is exacerbating the problem, but they are either unwilling or somehow unable to stop. In other words, his behavior causes her criticism causes his anger, resulting in a never-ending libido-lowering downward spiral. The following 47-year-old woman identified as having a partner who was extremely angry. Her husband has "gained a significant amount of weight and refuses to lose it," and, instead of being intimate, "he'd rather be on the Internet and watch TV at the same time." We asked her, in an online interview, to try and explain why she thought he was so angry.

He says that I'm "too controlling and always right." Too critical might better describe it. He isn't as detail oriented as I am, so he gets annoyed when I have to redo something he did, like clean the bathroom. When we're cleaning up after dinner, he leaves before we're finished—my standards of cleanliness are higher than his. I always clean up after myself in the bathroom (wipe down the sink and mirror) but he refuses to do so. He says "he forgets."

One partner is often neater than the other, and, at the risk of being stereotypical, it's usually the female. This can, of course, be approached with humor instead of derision and discussed rationally with an attempt at achieving détente. The degree of significance attached to not doing a perfect job cleaning the kitchen sink, or putting the cap back on the toothpaste tube, is likely to be in direct proportion to other marital issues of far greater importance. Anger at the trivial can mask anger at things too painful to explore, just as constantly refusing to comply with the easy stuff, like wiping off a bathroom counter, can indicate suppressed hostility, and purposeful annoyance. It can be a way to start a much desired fight, something to throw a pail of water on passion before it can even catch fire. When she complains to him of his negligence, here's what she says happens:

It inevitably disintegrates into him yelling and leaving the room, saying something like "Forget it. I can't win."

But how does she *really* feel?

His behavior, his negative attitude, his passive aggressiveness, and his lack of spontaneous affection . . . Well—I don't want to have sex with him, either!

Boy Meets Computer

His addiction to porn meant more to him than me and our marriage. He stopped having sex with me, but *I* would find him on a porn site almost every weekend morning, when we could have been making love. I just don't get it. What is it about men and porn? **(Female, 40s)**

Pornography is ubiquitous, and we've established that some male respondents are just saying yes to solitary sex—exclusively—and many female respondents believe the computer to be a serious rival for their husband's erotic attention. Sometimes porn is blamed for a sexless relationship, allowing serious physical or psychological issues to be left unexplored. This is not to suggest that all men who use porn online or elsewhere stop having sex with their wives. But sadly, often the Internet not only augments the real thing, it replaces it.

It was very hurtful to understand he preferred pornography to me and that was why we had sex so infrequently. **(Female, 53)**

She may have hit upon an inconvenient truth about her husband's preference for pornography over partnered sex, and it may not have anything to do with how she looks. It might be his way of maintaining emotional distance and avoiding intimacy. He's 56; he may have some performance anxiety he'd rather not deal with. Or he may find it a lot simpler and faster to focus only on his own pleasure.

We almost never have sex anymore. He seems addicted to pornography, and I really think he enjoys what is essentially just masturbation more than he ever enjoyed sex with me. I even tried watching with him, but I just didn't like it. **(Female, 36)**

This woman brings up the question of addiction. Addiction to online pornography is not a pathology recognized by the American Psychiatric Association. Some therapists say it doesn't exist; others believe it does. Some say it is abnormal behavior, but call it a compulsion, or poor impulse control. Whatever the label (and we, frankly, don't care), it's damaging to the preceding couple's marriage and life. It is positive that she attempted to watch with him, and also positive that she refused to continue watching when she realized it made her uncomfortable. It also indicates that he is open about what he is doing, which is preferable to being secretive. Alternatively, she may be using his passion for pornography to diffuse other issues in their marriage. This allows her to escape responsibility for his loss of desire.

> He waits to go on these sites until after I leave the house or go to bed. He told me he doesn't have a high sex drive, but that has to be false given the frequency he goes to porn sites. (Female, 30)

This woman concludes that her husband is lying when he says he doesn't have a high sex drive, because he visits erotic sites, secretly, on a regular basis. Sadly, she's correct—he is interested in sex, or at least orgasms, just not with her.

Thirty-nine percent of our female respondents reported that their husbands watched pornography online, 27 percent that their husbands masturbated while online, and 27 percent believed they masturbated without visual stimulation. These figures may all overlap. Clearly, some men are fueling their masturbatory fantasies in a variety of ways, or their wives think they are.

Online or off, it's all jealousy provoking and difficult to accept. It can be painfully uncomfortable for a woman to imagine her partner furtively performing acts of solitary sex instead of making love to her, focusing on a porn actress, centerfold, or some girl with a video cam, people who are willing to perform acts in public that she probably wouldn't dream of doing in private. The two quotes that follow are representative of many:

> I just can't compete with the bodies of the airbrushed women in the magazines. (Female, 44; husband, 45; married fifteen years)

> I have always felt insulted and demeaned by porn. He's in love with his "girls under the bed" (that's what I call his magazines) and I can't compete. (Female, 59; husband, 55; married twenty-five years)

A 57-year-old woman married to her 58-year-old husband for thirty-four years writes that her husband masturbates online and off-line, with videos, magazines, and DVDs. Pornography has always been an issue, she says, and it makes her "seethe," especially since a lot of it is "hard-core and revolting." She believes it has "desensitized him" and made him incapable of enjoying or even wanting to make love to her.

Clearly, if a man is masturbating on a regular basis, he likely has little or no desire or ability to also have partnered sex. His neglected spouse perceives him as selfish and lazy—unwilling to make an effort to please anyone but himself. However, there are often other things that are stopping him as well.

I Believe He Suffers from ED . . .

> . . . but he will not even ask his doctor about any possible help, and I have virtually begged him to do this. I am at a loss as to how this can be remedied, because he is a good man and I love

him, but two and a half years without sex is two and a half years too long. (Female, 50, married three years)

The woman in the preceding quote has described a man so embarrassed by impotence that he would rather sacrifice a sexual relationship with his wife than admit ED to his physician. He is not alone. The following respondent describes a similar situation:

Men seem to need to protect their ego in this area, but in doing so, they risk making their wives feel unloved and angry. It is such a shame that men will literally let their marriage fall into ruin just to protect their own feelings. They need to know that women, as nurturers, will understand anything except callous indifference to their love. To women, relationships are EVERYTHING! And there is no relationship that cannot be helped with open communication and compassion. (Female, 50s)

Few things, if any, can stop a guy from being sexual as surely as his inability to get an erection. This can be an exasperating conundrum for his wife, because why wouldn't he simply take a pill and get back to being "normal"? Is it that he prefers it this way? Isn't it really her age, looks, weight, wardrobe, job, or life?

Impotence can be the ultimate deal breaker in a relationship if a man is convinced that marital happiness (or his own) depends on his ability to get an erection.

Thirty-nine percent of the female respondents believe that their spouses suffer from erectile dysfunction, and of that group, 69 percent said no, their husbands did not seek any medical help. Men with this issue frequently shut down completely, refusing to discuss it with their physician, choosing solitary over partnered sex (no erection necessary), or no sex at all. Some fight just to avoid closeness, or become depressed, or pretend to be too tired. And some just flat out refuse, like the 52-year-old woman who told us that her 57-year-old husband pushed her hand away when she tried to touch him, whispering: "It doesn't work."

A woman in her 30s found something that did work, although we're not necessarily recommending it. After asking her husband to seek medical help for more than five years, she finally told him she was unhappy enough to be considering a trial separation. She said he finally went to the doctor, although she added, "I really think ED was a good excuse to stop having sex." She may be right, or her spouse may have been so embarrassed about his problem he preferred to pretend it didn't exist, until he realized the high price he might have to pay for his denial.

The following 54-year-old woman has been dating her 51-year-old boyfriend for four years. This is the second time around for them both—with each other—they were previously married for twelve years. She says:

One of the reasons we divorced was because of my dissatisfaction with our sex life. He says he is not gay, not having an affair, and I don't think he looks at porn. He has always been shy and somewhat repressed sexually. I think our situation is somewhat more complicated than most.

While answering the survey, she realizes:

It has just occurred to me that he stopped trying to make love to me after I asked him if he would talk to our doctor about getting medication for ED. I also bought him some L-Arginine because I read that it helps. He has not talked to the doctor and he has stopped approaching me completely.

She is correct that this is a complicated situation. Her current boyfriend/former husband may love her but have a combination of problems preventing him from physically expressing his love. (Based on her information, this may include low libido, fear of intimacy, depression, undisclosed trauma, and, clearly, erectile dysfunction.) Or he just may not want to be alone and is afraid of starting over. He surely wants to avoid revealing his issues to somebody new; he won't even talk to a doctor. We question what is keeping our female respondent in this dysfunctional relationship. It may be love, but she may also be afraid of being alone or beginning a new relationship, comfortable only when she considers herself victimized, or simply as sexually avoidant as her partner. After all, this time around she was fully aware of his low level of desire.

Impotence can be the ultimate deal breaker in a relationship if a man is convinced that marital happiness (or his own) depends on his ability to get an erection. The following 53-year-old woman has been in a serious relationship with her 50-year-old boyfriend for two years, but says it may end soon. He is impotent and will not get medical help for it. She poignantly explains:

He cannot make a commitment because he feels less than a man due to his sexual problem. I feel that men allow sexual problems to ruin a lot of really good relationships. Men do not have a clue about women and what they truly want. I want the companionship, and if the sex comes normally, that's great; but if it doesn't, then we can satisfy our needs in other ways. Men think that if intercourse is not achievable that it is just no good for the lady. I just want him for the great guy he is and all that he does for me otherwise.

He No Longer Finds Me Attractive

It's very hard for me to believe that men find me attractive, even though the mirror tells me differently. Being repeatedly turned down has been very hard on my self-esteem. It is hard not to see myself in his eyes. **(Female, 37)**

If many men base their self-worth on their bank account and their potency, many women base it on their looks and dress size. They have every reason to do so. We live in a culture that worships money, beauty, fame, and youth. A rich husband, a pretty wife—these are ultimate status symbols. What makes this so difficult, for almost everyone, is that extraordinary beauty, immense wealth, and superstar fame are extremely rare. The one prize we all have at one time is youth, but it's gone almost before we realize its value, and all the Botox and surgery in the world can do no more than pretend it's not. Times are changing, of course. Today, more women are in graduate school than men, and these executives, entrepreneurs, lawyers, and doctors of the future may feel differently about the male wealth/female beauty equation. But, for now, most women want to be young, attractive, and slim, or, like this 56-year-old female, long for their husbands to develop a pragmatic appreciation of what they've got: "I wish our society educated men to accept the aging of their women and how to cherish growing old together and not idolize youth. We were young and enjoyed it. Now we can enjoy aging."

One female respondent, 44, clearly illustrated how important self-perceived body image can be when she described this traumatic incident in her marriage. One afternoon she walked into the bedroom and found her husband in bed with another woman. To compound this terrible situation, her children, and the other woman's children, were in the family room downstairs while all this was going on. What did this traumatized wife do next? She checked out how her body compared with the competition: "She was the same weight as me, so I know that wasn't the reason this happened."

Forty percent of the women in our survey felt that they were no longer attractive to their husbands; 28 percent believed the reason was excess weight. (However, only 10 percent thought that losing weight would restore their husband's libido.) A 30-year-old wife explained away her 35-year-old husband's lack of sexual desire for her by saying, simply: "I gained weight. I don't look the way I used to look; therefore, he is not attracted to me." They've been married for only two years.

> He said he had to picture other women in his mind to climax. I think it is because I started to age. I can't not age. I think he would desire me if I had a firm, young, sexy body. It is like it turns him off to have to touch me or even look at me. **(Female, 54)**

The 59-year-old husband of the woman in the preceding quote has resorted to cruel and sadistic remarks in order to prevent being sexually or emotionally close with the woman he has been married to for thirty-three years. Although it is not possible to determine why he no longer desires her, or what is causing his anger, it seems clear that he is blaming his wife for his difficulty achieving orgasm or maintaining an erection. His body, of course, is five years older than hers, which might be distressing him more than he cares to admit, even to himself.

The 44-year-old woman quoted next is now divorced from her 38-year-old husband, who had an affair. She thinks the sex stopped, and maybe even the affair started, because "I gained weight, which he finds unattractive." She says that if she could do things differently, she would: "pay attention to who I married. If he is going to be turned off by a twenty-pound weight gain, he's very shallow. I thought there was more to what we had."

The following woman (35) is aware that her husband (38) has severe intimacy problems—and had them with his previous partners, too—and yet she blames herself for his inappropriate behavior when she says:

"I can't help but believe I am physically unattractive. Why else would he want to chat with other women online and have phone sex with them?"

It is difficult for many women to comprehend that their partners think they are desirable, but still choose not to be intimate.

The woman correctly identifies her husband's fear of intimacy. That's why he's so comfortable chatting online and having phone sex with anonymous, emotionally disposable partners, but not making love to his wife. And yet, she still blames her appearance for his infidelities. It is difficult for many women to comprehend that their partners think they are desirable, but still choose not to be intimate. This man may have such a strong fear of abandonment that he thinks anonymous relationships and masturbatory fantasies are his best option, or a buffer zone against the unimaginable pain of his wife leaving him. Sadly, without help, he may lose her.

And a woman in her 20s, married to a man in his 40s, says that she gained "what he considers to be a lot of weight," and that's why he stopped making love to her, although "he has lost all his hair, and has gained fifty-plus pounds." She adds: "I'm the undesirable one?"

He's Having an Affair

Fidelity is ingrained into most women's thinking when it comes to marriage. It goes with the territory, therefore, that when a man stops being sexual with his wife, "he must be cheating" often is the first thing that comes to mind. Sometimes the affair isn't imaginary, there is proof. However, as we mentioned previously, the infidelity rate of men in sexless marriages is about the national average of men in all marriages, around 20 percent. Thus, fidelity does not indicate a passionate marriage, and infidelity is not, in any way, a guaranteed result of a sexless one. Most men (and most women) don't stray.

You don't need us to tell you that infidelity is something you want to avoid, and even if only one in five men said they're unfaithful, that may be great for the other four women, but not for you if you suspect, or know for certain, your guy is the fifth.

The infidelity rate of men in sexless marriages is about the national average of men in all marriages, around 20 percent.

There are few things more painful than betrayal by someone you love, and it is worth trying to prevent in any way you possibly can. If your marriage is devoid of intimacy, it is imperative that you talk about it, and listen hard to each other. If you are certain of infidelity, we urge you to talk to each other, listen to each other, and, if you feel you need professional help, get it immediately. It really is possible to emerge a stronger, better couple once all the reasons for the infidelity are revealed. This isn't just sententious psychobabble; it really is possible to become stronger as a couple, but not without a lot of honesty, love, and work.

He Never Wanted Sex

Twenty-eight percent of the women who responded to our survey reported that intimacy ended prior to or in the first year of marriage, and 19 percent suggested that although sex may have occurred on occasion, it was never a priority for their partners, agreeing that "he wasn't interested in sex to begin with." Some believed things would get better with time. Others were so much in love, or so anxious to marry, that they ignored what was clearly evident. As one 53-year-old woman said:

Within the first month he started avoiding sex and me. Generally sex happened every two or three months. This was the norm for sixteen years. Five years ago, after nine months of abstinence, I approached him and he pushed me away and told me to leave him alone. I am hurt. I have not had sex with him or anyone else in five years.

Other women who were aware of their partners' lack of interest in sex from the start made the mistake of thinking that marriage, somehow, would transform their men into passionate lovers. A 37-year-old told us that she thought "all he needed was some normalcy and structure." A 32-year-old said: "There was very little sex even during our courtship, but I was young and naïve enough to believe marriage and a good home would improve the situation. Needless to say, it only became worse."

For some women, there is some comfort in learning that their husband has a low libido; as reasons go, it can be less painful than, say, infidelity. A 40-year-old woman responded to a survey question by writing:

He always had a reason, even in the beginning. [He would say] "I'm having a hard time at work, I'm stressed and I'm tired." It was never the right time. Nor was it ever spontaneous, where we could steal away in the bedroom for five minutes.

In a follow-up interview, she mentioned that she and her husband went into counseling, separately and together, during the last three years of their marriage. (They are now divorced.) Privately, she asked if the therapist believed her husband was gay or having an affair. The therapist told her she thought her husband was asexual, just not that interested in lovemaking. That came as a sense of relief. As she stated: ". . . it wasn't about me." The relief was, naturally, bittersweet: "At the same time, there was nothing I could do about it."

PART II

inside the sexless man's mind

three

NOT TONIGHT, DEAR,
WE'RE MARRIED

Here's something that surprised us a lot. Twenty-eight percent of the women said that their partners stopped being sexual with them almost at once, that the intimacy ended either before the marriage (10%), on the honeymoon (3%), or during the first year (15%). The men's numbers weren't nearly as high. Only 9 percent of male respondents said they stopped being sexual during, or before, the first year of marriage. Some marriages seem to be destined for celibacy. But here's something else that surprised us: more than 70 percent of these marriages remained intact.

Why is it that many men no longer see their spouses as desirable so soon after commitment?

Often women in this situation told us that sex was frequent and impassioned at first, but then mysteriously, and abruptly, ended. The following 43-year-old woman told us her 51-year-old spouse stopped being sexual in the first year of marriage. They've been married for three years.

It's odd . . . before we married and during the start of the first year of marriage, my husband would initiate sex, tell me how beautiful I was, participate in oral sex and try many different positions and even places. Now he doesn't like sex and refuses to participate in oral at all. I've tried to talk to him in a noncon- frontational way. He just says that he's tired and his blood pressure medication has affected his sex drive.

A 30-year-old woman who cohabited with her partner for twelve years before they got married states:

The minute I became his wife I feel he stopped seeing me as a sexual being. He told me wives do not dress in sexy underwear, etc. I am only thirty years old and feel a part of me has died. I believe in the marriage vows, but within a year of marriage I was thinking about divorce, due to the stress of my husband not wanting me.

Sometimes a man changes his sexual behavior as soon as he mar- ries, because the woman is no longer a girlfriend, or someone to share what he secretly, even subconsciously, considers to be illicit sex. Now she's a wife, and sex is suddenly both sanctioned and a job. It's just not exciting anymore. As one 42-year-old woman put it: "Girlfriends are okay to have sex with, but if that girlfriend becomes your wife, suddenly you are sullying her by making love."

The madonna/whore syndrome refers to men who see women as either hotties or homemakers, but never both. A woman is either re- spectable and "good," or sexy and "bad." A man who relates to women this way may end intimacy as soon as his girlfriend and he decide to get married. Passionate sex, although appropriate for a ca- sual relationship, is impossible in a committed one. The couple dis- cussed in the following quote didn't have sex when they were married, but did after they divorced, lived in different towns, and resumed a dating relationship.

> He was very sexually active prior to marriage, but a few weeks before the wedding he started to lose interest. We didn't consummate our marriage until six months later. Then it was about three to six times per year, until the sixth year when sex stopped completely until, after ten years of marriage, we divorced. After the divorce he moved to another town, but we would have sex every weekend when he visited. He is now remarried. **(Female, 58)**

The next quote is from a 53-year-old woman who has been married to her 54-year-old husband for twenty-seven years, but has been separated for the past three:

> We are currently separated with the main reason being lack of interest in sex and passion on his part. As soon as we married, the relationship went from being all about sex to him being infrequently interested, at least with me. The only time he showed his former interest was when I said I was in love with someone else and wanted a divorce. I am very glad you're researching this issue. I always felt alone in this. Most of my friends complained of husbands wanting sex all the time!

It is likely that this woman's husband had such a strong fear of intimacy that he felt the marriage would consume him unless he protected himself. He was fine until the wedding day, when, like a little boy who holds his breath to defy his parents, he withheld sex as a way to establish his freedom. He felt that this would protect him from pain if his wife ever left him. When the worst happened, and she said she was in love with another man and wanted a divorce, his libido returned.

She was no longer his wife, but a woman to be wooed and won all over again. Hormones kicked in, keeping him frequently aroused in order to recapture her affection and make her his wife once more.

Crisis sometimes allows people to do some sexual time travel, and return, albeit briefly, to when they first met and fell in love. That's what happened here. We think, however, that the passion would have stopped if she decided to abandon her new lover and remain married. As inexplicably as the excitement returned, it would have deserted him once more.

Some men may have perfectly normal libidos, but psychological issues prevent them from having a close intimate relationship.

WHY ELSE WOULD THE PASSION END SO SOON?

In other chapters we will discuss the possibility of an asexual or homosexual man marrying because he wants love, companionship, social status, acceptance, and family, but not sex. These men, as well as men who have lower than average libidos, would tend to have little or no sex very shortly after marriage, or even before. Women would probably notice that these guys may be wonderful in other ways, but are just not very passionate.

Other men may have perfectly normal libidos, but psychological issues prevent them from having a close intimate relationship. If "abandoned" by one or both parents as a child due to death, mental or physical illness, or divorce, or if truly neglected by desertion, the fear of being rejected in this way again may prevent a man from ever allowing real intimacy. It is a terrible conflict: he loves his wife so much he can't possibly risk losing her, so he protects himself by avoiding the most committed thing he can do—having a fulfilling sexual relationship.

Almost 50 percent of the women said that their partners were angry and 52 percent said they were depressed. This was often in combination with physiological factors. Erectile dysfunction and difficulty reaching orgasm were mentioned numerous times by both men and women who say that sexual relations ended before, or right after, the wedding vows. Other men were on medication that lowered their libidos, and, in rare cases, had medical reasons why sex was not feasible.

It is possible that men severely suffering from these psychological and physiological issues, especially if in combination with loss of libido, are more likely to stop being sexual with their wives as soon as they feel confident they can do so and still hold on to the relationship. Depending on the couple, this can be right after moving in together, or soon after the wedding day.

We had a difficult time finding any literature or studies focusing on marriages that are sexually inactive from the start, but our respondents gave us many valuable insights. We have divided this rapid decline or complete absence of intimacy into three parts—during the engagement (other than those who for religious or moral reasons wait until marriage to consummate a relationship), on the honeymoon, and during the first year. We'll listen to the men first.

It Ended Before the Wedding Day

Men Explain Why

Of the few male respondents who reported stopping all sexual contact with their wives prior to the wedding, the majority mentioned erectile dysfunction and/or inability to reach orgasm. Perhaps to diffuse some of the responsibility, they also say that their partners are "not sexually adventurous" (something we will explore in chapter 5). In these cases, how would they know? Their ages range from 45 to 61.

The following quote is from a 48-year-old man who has been married for eighteen years. In addition to his problem of inhibited ejaculation (inability to attain orgasm), he says he is angry at his wife because she is controlling. He also mentions that she is not his "physical type." He watches pornography online and on videos, and he has had an affair.

I suffer from inhibited ejaculation when in a committed relationship. I was happy when I was single because as soon as the sexual dysfunction started I would simply move on to a new person. This would usually happen after two or three encounters. I can't do that in my marriage. I am very sad that I am unable to have sex with my wife because I do care for her. I really thought sex therapy would help, but I have visited many therapists and they haven't been able to resolve the problem.

Although men sometimes experience inhibited ejaculation (15% of the men who responded to our survey said they did), this is usually a side effect of medication or street drugs such as cocaine and heroin. However, this man writes that the problem *only* occurs when he's in a committed relationship. When single, as long as he was in a noncommitted relationship, he was able to climax. He appears to want the security and love of an emotionally intimate relationship, since he has "visited many therapists" without success. He is also so scared of intimacy, he is making sure that his marriage has as little as possible. Clearly, he is withholding something he considers to be precious. Perhaps he truly hasn't found a therapist able to help him, or he just finds a new one at the first sign of unpleasant issues revealed. However, for some additional reasons not to be intimate, he still manages to blame his wife for being controlling, and even for not being his physical type.

Another man, 61, has been married to his 52-year-old spouse for one year. He incongruously shifts all responsibility for not being intimate by saying that she is not sexually adventurous and doesn't enjoy lovemaking: "Sex is unimportant to her, but very important to me. She has little or no libido." He also suffers from inhibited ejaculation.

A 45-year-old man told us his 43-year-old wife of eighteen years was lacking in sexual adventure, and that he watches a considerable amount of pornography. He also said: "I am not turned on by my wife and suffer severe orgasmic difficulties and mild erectile dysfunction that makes sex unpleasant and stressful." What does he expect the future to be like? "We will remain sexless until one of us dies."

Although women's difficulty attaining orgasm seems to be a ubiquitous topic, male-inhibited orgasm is not written about a lot. And yet, 27 percent of the women thought it was a reason their husbands stopped being sexual with them.

Another 54-year-old man, married for thirty-four years to his 54-year-old wife, said that the problem was due to a lack of desire on his part: "I lost my libido and I'm not sure why. I do take blood pressure medication." But he also mentions that his wife is not sexually adventurous.

Women Tell What They Think Happened

We mostly stopped having sex before we were married. His belief is that sex is a good way to get to know someone, but useless after that. (Female, 50s)

Of the numerous women who said that sex either stopped or dramatically declined prior to marriage (but they decided to wed, anyway), more than half reported that their husbands were angry and depressed, and many said that their spouses suffered from ED.

Some got married because they believed things would improve; others said that sex wasn't too important—companionship was their main priority. One woman, 28, put it this way:

> I don't think we have a bad marriage; sex is not the only thing.
> It would be better if we had it more, but I'm still happy.

This woman is trying hard to adjust and accept. She's young, and so is her spouse, who is 30. She says he neither is taking medication that lowers his libido nor is depressed, and she doesn't suspect infidelity. She has no explanation except that her husband doesn't care very much about sex. She may be right.

We admire this woman's maturity. She was probably aware that her sexual needs were a bit, but not too much, stronger than his from the start. She married him anyway, and is focusing on the good in the relationship and the man, rather than trying to turn him into something he's not.

A 58-year-old woman says of her 51-year-old husband of three years:

> He wasn't sexual to begin with and with his heart condition and
> the medications, sex has really been lacking. We have a good
> relationship; it just lacks sex.

Obviously, this woman was aware that her marriage wasn't going to be very sexual, although her husband's health issues and medications intensified the situation. A "good relationship" is impossible without love, kindness, and understanding, which they seem to have. Hopefully, her husband's lack of desire and inability to be sexual does not preclude them being physical with each other—touching, holding hands, and kissing. A lack of physical contact can be more devastating to a marriage than a lack of sex.

It is also quite possible that she is content, at this time of her life, to be in this type of marriage, and her husband's condition allows her to be, without pressure from him to change.

Another woman, 51, said that her 56-year-old husband suffered from inhibited ejaculation, ED, and depression, and he was taking medication that diminished his sex drive. Nevertheless, she says that an "open" marriage allows them to thrive.

> My husband suffers from chronic pain that is exacerbated by most sexual activities. Our relationship is consensually open and he is friends with my other lovers. We are happy together.

The polyamorous (multiple-partnered or "open") marriage that this woman is describing is clearly not for most. Although the lack of available partners has resulted in certain cultures encouraging marriage between a man and several women, a culture where a female has several husbands is far rarer. This is because, historically, the reason for multiple partners was propagation of the species, and women can give birth once a year, at most. A harem, however, can allow one male to father many offspring.

The concept of multiple marriage (or emotionally committed) partners is generally condemned in our society and has been illegal since the nineteenth century. The very idea of a spouse having a sexual relationship with someone else is (usually) a threat to our most primal needs—the survival of the family, and our own feelings of security and self-worth.

This couple has chosen it as a way of life—the key to keeping their marriage intact and a far more honest choice than infidelity. But why so many partners? There may be safety in numbers; the fact that she has many lovers might be easier for her husband to accept than just one special companion.

A 28-year-old who identified herself as "intensely sexual" has not yet married her fiancé, also 28. He suffers from ED but has not seen a urologist. She intends to go through with the wedding in spite of his being "not a very sexual person, and shy."

The woman we just quoted is not about to walk down the aisle; she's about to march through a minefield. She's highly sexual; he's not.

He suffers from ED, but won't see a doctor. And, by the way, she never mentions love. What's remarkable is his refusal to try and solve a problem that is unlikely to disappear after marriage, and her acceptance of the situation. Why is she going through with this marriage? We can only speculate, but he might have something she wants, like power or money, that makes sexual compatibility less important. Or her "intense" sexuality may give her what she perceives as an upper hand. She may see his ED as insurance against infidelity.

Some women told us that a life without sex
was preferable to living alone.

Others told us, with honesty and clarity, that a life without sex was preferable to living alone, even if it wasn't all they had hoped for. As a 59-year-old woman married to her husband (53) for three years put it:

> I know there's a lot to be said for pure companionship, but that's not what I was looking for. He is a good husband for the most part. I feel that I'm too old to be on my own or go out and find someone else.

And sometimes, with a combination of effort and patience, the story can have a happy ending. The following woman's does. She's 45, her husband is 53. They didn't have intercourse before marriage, because he told her things such as: "I am very nervous because I haven't had sex in three years." She loved him, he loved her, and they married anyway. When things didn't improve, she initially blamed herself. "I took all the responsibility for not having sex. I thought it was because I wasn't fashion-magazine beautiful, or thin, or not creative enough." After two years of this, she decided to try and improve the situation, ultimately learning that her appearance had nothing what-soever to do with the problem, which turned out to be hormonal. His testosterone was significantly below normal. She expresses the reso-lution to their problem with eloquence:

> It took a great deal of research and insistence to get him to go to a urologist specializing in sexual dysfunction. It was diag-nosed that he had very low testosterone, which not only ac-counted for his ED, but his lack of energy, low sex drive, and depression. His urologist literally saved our marriage from be-coming "roommates with a joint bank account." He is now healthy and sexually dynamic, thanks to hormone replacement therapy and the judicious use of an erectile enhancement drug. He and I are enjoying a honeymoon phase in the third year of our relationship. If I had been surer of myself, this could have happened on our actual honeymoon. I think that women have to stop feeling that they are the sole focus of their mate's sex drive.

We applaud this woman's bravery and tenacity, and we admire her husband's courage, too. He was willing to talk, listen, and find a solution and to put his wife's needs ahead of his possible embarrass-ment.

Those first conversations, after she decided she wanted more and would try to improve the intimate side of their lives, must have been difficult. After all, she had married him accepting that the relation-ship would likely be platonic, and he had no reason to expect things to change. She was able to shift her thinking away from herself, and with the support of her partner and their physician, find a solution. A testosterone level that is low enough to cause her husband's symp-toms is rare, as we discuss in chapter 11. But it can happen. Neuro-chemistry is a young science, and there are still numerous unanswered questions. This respondent puts it well:

It is such a complex thing, this commingling of the emotional, mental, and physical that makes up our sexuality. There should be much more open, honest talking about it.

WHY SOME MEN SAY "I WON'T" AFTER SAYING "I DO"

Fourteen men, ranging in age from 24 to 72, said that there was no honeymoon period to their marriage; the sex stopped immediately after taking the vows. In all cases of this limited sample, the guys reported that their wives were not sexually adventurous and didn't seem to enjoy sex, and all said that they themselves were angry. The following 46-year-old man is about to leave his wife of twenty-two years:

> My wife has no interest in sex. Never has. Both of us were churchgoing virgins when we got married. Ten years ago, she decided she wanted children and she directed the sex, of course, to eventually have our family. The sex was clinical and I don't remember it. My wife and I are like brother and sister. I feel a lot of anger toward her that I suppress. I am having an affair now and will be leaving my marriage for another woman— a real woman. Finally, I am wanted and desired. I am salvaging what is left of my manhood. I feel like I am waking up after too long a sleep and it is wondrous. I had no idea how great a blow job feels!

This couple started out with an advantage in that they shared the same points of view about religion and premarital sex. However, they seem to have abstained from conversation, too. They should have discussed their feelings about how important a role, if any, they wanted sex to play in their married life. From what he writes, it appears that his wife believed that sex was for procreation only, and they didn't consummate the marriage until, twelve years later, it was time to start a family. All he remembers about this is that he doesn't remember it.

Now, at the age of 46, he's having his first real sexual experience with a woman who seems to enjoy both lovemaking and him. He is filled with joy, preparing to leave his wife and children and begin a new life with a partner who believes in premarital sex (even with a married man). We assume his religious beliefs have shifted. Although his previous relationship might have appeared to have a strong foundation in the beginning, serious issues were never discussed. Things that made him angry were "suppressed" along with his sex drive. The downfall of this marriage was caused by everything that was never said.

The next man was 24 years old when he married his 24-year-old bride. Similar to the man we just quoted, they were in their early 20s when they married, and they had abstained from premarital sex and all intimate conversation. They are now divorced.

> She was a virgin when we married. I was taught to treat a woman with sensitivity and honor. She did not seem to crave me or sex in general, and whenever we would attempt intercourse, the image of me hurting her would cause me to lose my erection. I think it would have helped if she ever initiated sex, but she didn't. So I never felt desired, and that just added to the problem when we attempted intercourse. To make things worse, we never openly discussed what was going on and why. I'm not certain I would know how if I had the chance.

We asked him if he could do things over, what he would have done differently. His response is poignant. It centers on communicating with honesty, which might have saved their marriage.

1. Find the courage, and words, to talk to her about what was going on inside of me.

2. Seek counseling.
3. Ask her to take the initiative, sometimes.
4. Tell her I need to feel desired.
5. Work in counseling to discover and treat the core issues needing attention.
6. Not allow the two of us to drift apart and divorce.

WOMEN TRY TO UNDERSTAND WHY THE HONEYMOON WAS LEFT AT THE ALTAR

Young girls brought up on romance novels, fairy tales, and "happily ever after" imagine that their honeymoon will be a romantic, magical, passionate time. The night is expected to be a celebration of sex and love. The inexperienced and naïve (or those engaging in wishful thinking) may hope that marriage will finally make their nonresponsive partner passionate. It therefore can be a trauma when there is no intimacy on the honeymoon. The marriage may not be consummated, and the pain and disappointment can be too embarrassing to discuss with anyone. Many women think their situation is unique. As one 50-year-old woman, now divorced, said:

> I was really glad to see this survey and know it wasn't just me, that there are other women out there with husbands like mine.

A 33-year-old woman with two young children, married for ten years to her 35-year-old husband, wrote that she was determined to "kill her sexuality" to remain married and faithful. She called it the "sacrifice of a wife and mother." She was depressed, however, and said she felt her husband "cheated" her by not revealing his lack of desire prior to marriage. She had no way of knowing, since they decided not to have sex until after they were married.

---

*Abstinence may be a convenient way to cover up extreme
sexual repression, or a very low libido.*

We don't question remaining abstinent prior to marriage for
religious or moral reasons, any more than we would question premarital sex. These are deeply personal, religious, and spiritual decisions. However, we do strongly question those couples who choose
celibacy before marriage and also omit any discussions about what
they hope the intimate part of their lives will be like after the
wedding. Abstinence may be a convenient way to cover up extreme
sexual repression, or a very low libido.

Some women reported a lot of passion prior to the honeymoon,
when it suddenly came to a stop. This 51-year-old recently divorced
woman was married to her 52-year-old husband for thirty years:

> We were very sexually active prior to marriage. Once married, I
> think he saw me as his mother. Seven years later we had a child,
> and the sex totally ended. He has always hated his mother and
> projected angry feelings onto me. We are currently divorced.

When in their teens or early 20s, her future husband had no difficulty becoming aroused by a "bad" girl; that is, one willing to have sex
outside of marriage. After the wedding, intimacy was no longer exciting,
because the "bad" girl was now "good." Once that "good" girl became a
mother, the sex stopped completely. If he did, indeed, despise his mother,
this may have compounded his problem even more. It is amazing how
powerful this type of "good girl/bad girl" psychological scenario can be,
managing to suppress the passion of even very young men.

The following woman, 40, has been married to her 47-year-old
husband for six years:

I believe it was the chase. He pursued me with great determi-
nation; then, on the honeymoon, he lost interest. It was like a
conquest for him.

This is an interesting statement. If her husband wanted only a
"conquest," he probably would have "lost interest" either immediately after the first sexual encounter or after the wedding date was
set. Instead, he went through with the wedding, but had no desire to
make love to his new bride, not even on the honeymoon. This could
be yet another example of a guy unable to be aroused by a "good"
woman—his wife.

But there is something we haven't yet considered. It's possible for a
man to have such diminished self-esteem that he is unable to be attracted to a woman once she becomes his spouse, reminiscent of a
note Groucho Marx wrote to the Beverly Hills Country Club: "Please
accept my resignation. I don't want to belong to any club that will accept me as a member."

Intimacy Stopped in the First Year

Men Explain Why

Men who told us passion stopped not immediately, but in the first
year of marriage, ranged in age from 26 to 76 and had been married
for between one and twenty-six years. Conventional wisdom looks at
age and number of years married as contributing factors to decreased
libido in men and women, but this doesn't seem to be the case here.
The men who said that the sex stopped soon after marriage did have
a few things in common, however.

Many suffered from ED. A 53-year-old man who did said: "You
don't absolutely need sex to grow in life and love."

Another man, 37, first on medication with a libido-lowering side
effect and now suffering from impotence, is caught in a vortex of
negativity. His wife, 40, feels she is to blame for his erectile dysfunc-

tion and he can't convince her she isn't. They have been married for less than one year.

> Initially I was on the antidepressant Wellbutrin and that seemed to kill my drive. *[Note: Wellbutrin usually does not have a libido-lowering side effect.]* Then my wife started blaming herself, which put a lot of pressure on me to perform, and I had a lot of trouble getting and maintaining an erection. The main problem is when my wife gets very sad. All I can think of is I don't want to hurt her again. Viagra helps me but she thinks I'm too young to be on it and thinks I either need a pill or to be drinking to be with her. She doesn't understand it is a mental problem. I want to avoid the possibility of pain. I think we will stay married, but I think resentment will build in her and she will grow to hate me because I've been hurting her.

It is unfortunate that many women cannot separate themselves from their husband's problems of impotence. Chapter 8 explores this issue in greater depth, let us say here (again) that erectile dysfunction and wife are rarely related, and there is even less possibility of any connection in the first year of marriage. The above situation may have been averted, or at least improved, if the husband's physician educated the couple as to the way the prescribed medications work, deleterious effects that commonly occur, and possible alternatives.

Other men, not surprisingly, tossed the ball into their wife's court, saying that their spouses had little sense of adventure and didn't seem to enjoy sex. One man (52) married to his wife (48) for eleven years, said that the sex stopped immediately and completely because "her lack of interest made me stop." Another man (29) married for less than two years (his wife is 25) writes:

> My wife says birth control pills decreased her desire. I say something else killed her desire the same time she started

taking them. She gained a lot of weight. I don't care but I know she does. She hasn't tried to lose the weight. She signed up for a gym but has only gone twice.

Although our book is exploring why men stop being sexual with their partners, if a guy is consistently turned down, he may eventually just stop trying. This may be, at least to some extent, what happened here. Birth control pills can have a libido-lowering effect. This can be for physiological reasons (such as hormonal issues), or psychological ones (for example, she really wants to become pregnant, is angry her husband doesn't want her to, and is punishing him). It may be a combination of both. It is curious that he seems so certain that something else ended her desire that he isn't even suggesting they experiment with another method of birth control.

And another man (54) married to his wife (51) for twelve years says that he stopped having sex with her right after their marriage because: "She doesn't have an adventuresome approach. She rarely made the first move." Clearly, he didn't, either.

Women Tell Us What They Think Happened

Fifteen percent of the female respondents said that sex stopped in the first year of marriage. Although some were unsure of the reasons, many felt that libido-lowering drugs for a variety of diseases including high blood pressure, diabetes, OCD, and depression were the cause.

The following woman, 52, has been married to her 56-year-old husband for two years. Before the wedding, they had oral sex frequently, but never intercourse. After the honeymoon, all intimacy stopped. Her husband is impotent and tells her that his doctor won't prescribe Viagra because of other medication that he is taking. He refuses to seek alternative treatment, or to be sexual without an erection. She writes: "I can live without sex. I just wish he wouldn't give up, not even try."

This woman is understandably sad and confused about her

husband's reluctance to be sexual now that they are married, since his medical condition and ED did not prevent them from having an intimate life before. He is probably conflicted about the marriage and withholding all contact as a way to demonstrate this. Perhaps he is afraid that his wife will find a man to satisfy her sexually in ways he thinks he can't, and stopping all intimacy is a way of diffusing potential pain.

The following 45-year-old woman is married to a man, 53, whom she describes as angry and depressed, with a preference for online pornography. After two years of marriage, they have separated.

> I came with a young child, which had a tremendous impact on our relationship. My husband is an extremely unhappy person. His presence is toxic.

And the following woman, 64, has been married for four years to a man, 65, she describes as depressed. She is in therapy and says although she "loves him very much" she will leave unless he "gets it together." She continues:

> The excitement has disappeared, and the necessary creativity has not taken place. I'm not 16 anymore, but he ain't a teenager in body appearance, either. I haven't changed from the first few months when he couldn't get enough of me. Now he seems to think of it as "work." What a pity for both of us.

We agree that this is a pitiful situation, for a variety of reasons. Her husband may have been delighted to get back the intensity of desire that accompanies a new and loving relationship, and disappointed that it didn't last past the first few months, which is, in fact, often how long that kind of "excitement" does last, especially for a mature man. She is upset because she thinks he no longer wants her. However, she mentions he is depressed. This is probably lowering his libido, and certain antidepressants could be lowering it even more, and/or causing erectile dysfunction. Although she thinks it might have to do with the way she looks, and worries that he doesn't think she's sexy, this has nothing to do with her appearance. He was aware of her age and body type long before the wedding day and they've only been married for a few years. As far as "creativity" goes, it may well be lacking on both their parts. What really seems "a pity" is that she has given her marriage an expiration date, and he is unwilling to try and solve the problem.

WHY SEX STOPS SO SOON: AN ABUNDANCE OF POSSIBILITIES

Psychiatrist, sex therapist, and author Avodah Offit wrote: "Rather than being surprised at the reduction in sex drive, I am surprised that any remains at all in people bound to one another for better or for worse. So much in life is worse." But Offit is not speaking of that magical first year when newlyweds believe that better is all there is.

Many of the respondents who claim that sex stopped almost immediately seem to be on medications that are decreasing their sex drive. (It is imperative that side effects of all medications be discussed with your physician. There may be alternative drugs that do not lower the libido.) Others suffer from ED, but don't seek help, and prefer instead to avoid sex completely. The majority of women report men who are angry and depressed. This could be caused, at least in part, by anticipated humiliation. Then there are the women who pretend to orgasm, perhaps fearful of bruising their partners' not yet married egos. When they finally decide to confess, the truth may end the passion. Some men may fear an unwanted pregnancy, no matter how unrealistic. We can assume that some simply find sex unnecessary, or frightening; it just might provide more pain than pleasure. Intimacy is a risky thing. It may be easier to show passion to a transitory lover; there is no fear of loss or abandonment. Once the ultimate commitment of marriage comes along, the stakes seem to suddenly be too high.

SOMETIMES, WATER SEEKS ITS OWN LEVEL

A 40-year-old woman who has been in a sexless marriage from the very start, which was eleven years ago, is currently thinking about getting a divorce. She told us that her husband has always avoided intimacy in his life, with her and everyone else. But neither she, nor any other woman, said that a lack of intimacy would suit her just fine, although in some cases this certainly must be true. Some women, when faced with a marriage destined to be without passion from the beginning, must secretly think it a good thing. Often, those with a fear of intimacy and attachment look for others with similar qualities.

four

PREGNANCY AND THE
END OF PASSION

It is not uncommon for a man to both welcome the idea of becoming a new father and feel ambivalence once pregnancy is confirmed. It will soon no longer be just him and his partner, and to be more specific, he probably won't be her top priority for the next eighteen years. Some day soon his girlfriend is going to turn into a mommy. A first child is an ending as well as a beginning; some men perceive it as an end of the innocence. The sense of impending responsibility can be overwhelming.

And then there's the sex act itself. Certain positions are difficult. He can be terrified of hurting his wife or unborn baby. And although some men find a third-trimester woman beautiful, others don't. For example, one 44-year-old man wrote that he stopped being sexual with his spouse six years ago when she was pregnant with their son: "The thought of sex during pregnancy was somehow quite unappealing, and after the baby was born I never got back to trying again."

Few issues are more important to discuss prior to marriage than whether or not a couple wants to have children.

Even if a man isn't a first-time father, the uncertainty of having more children may be temporarily shutting down his libido. If she wants another and he doesn't, not being sexual can be a way to express his anger and frustration.

There are men who have such a strong fear of becoming a parent, they avoid sex. A 47-year-old woman, unlikely to conceive, told us her 63-year-old husband has completely stopped being intimate with her when her physician told her she had to stop taking the pill, the only birth control method he considers reliable. They have been married for less than one year.

A 29-year-old woman, married for six years to her 49-year-old husband, had a similar problem, which was revealed in counseling:

He finally agreed to therapy and I was elated. The therapist, noticing the large difference in our ages, asked if I wanted children. I do, very much, and he always knew this, but he confessed that he really doesn't but was afraid to tell me, so he just stopped making love to me. (He knew I was no longer taking birth control pills.) The therapist suggested that he might have considered this would be a problem before he married someone so much younger than himself, and also that this was a very serious situation and needed to be resolved if the marriage was to survive. We made an appointment for the following week, but he canceled it without even discussing it with me. I think the only solution is a divorce. I find myself fantasizing about being single all the time.

Few issues are more important to discuss prior to marriage than whether or not a couple wants to have children. If they adamantly disagree about this, there is little chance that the marriage will be successful. Some people make the mistake of avoiding deal-breaking issues, but this woman didn't do that. She was clear about wanting a family from the start. Unfortunately, her partner either changed his mind when faced with the reality of becoming a new father in his 50s, or he lied, hoping he could wish it all away. Now he is bullying her and canceling appointments because their therapist is saying things he doesn't want his wife to hear, and he doesn't want to admit.

We have written quite a lot about communication. No two people will ever agree on everything, or want all of the same things, and needs change over time. Honestly and empathetically discussing these differences is the ideal. When honesty and empathy are missing, however, conversation is pointless. This woman thought she was expressing what was of primary importance to her in a marriage, and her fiancé concurred. He told her what she wanted to hear. We think it is an unfortunate example of someone being less than truthful to get what he wants most, ignoring the fact that it will probably, ultimately, cause him to lose it all.

THE SEXLESS STEPFATHER

Women with children from previous marriages told us that the tremendous responsibility of suddenly becoming stepfathers was enough to shut their husbands down sexually. This can be especially true of men who have no prior experience in parenting—the anxiety can be a libido killer. A 47-year-old woman told us that she thinks her husband stopped being sexual with her because he is so angry about being a "new" stepfather; he had no idea how difficult it would be. He is also resentful, she says, that she's no longer his "dream girl" now that they're all living together as a family. A 40-year-old woman wrote about a similar experience:

> Things were normal before the wedding...sex a couple of times a week. On the honeymoon, I took some sexy lingerie, which he liked, and everything was fine. After the wedding he moved in with me and my 9-year-old daughter and everything

changed. I wore the sexy stuff for him, and he was unable to perform and sometimes wouldn't even try. I scheduled special romantic nights for us when my daughter was away, and he either couldn't perform or wasn't interested. If I initiate sex, he feels pressured and can't perform. If he initiates sex, he feels pressured and can't perform. He says he gets excited but is afraid of failing so he can't perform. Eventually, I threw away the sexy lingerie and gave up on the romantic evenings. **(Female, 40, married one and a half years)**

A man may be suddenly sexually unresponsive to a woman after marrying her, if she is a mother and her children are now living with them. This may seem irrational; he knew what their lives would be like. But knowing it isn't living it, and these guys are suddenly facing responsibilities they were clearly not emotionally prepared for. There might be resentment about the situation—toward their wife, her children, or the children's father. They may be angry. She may not seem so accessible anymore. This can also happen if a woman marries a man whose young children are living with him. Suddenly, she's not just his adorable fiancée, she's a mom.

MOMMY NOT-SO-DEAREST

Sometimes passion continues until the woman becomes pregnant or gives birth, then stops abruptly. We are not talking about the drop in sexual frequency most new parents experience due to time constraints and exhaustion, which is to be expected, when the father of a newborn still desires his wife, but passion just has to be put on hold for a while. In a healthy relationship, pretty soon new parents get a babysitter, go away for the weekend, leave the child with Grandma and Grandpa—do whatever it takes. (And even so, sex may still be less frequent than it was before the baby.) What we are discussing here is quite different. Suddenly, a wife has become a mother, and it's no longer possible for her husband to perceive her as a sexual being.

Some men complained that they didn't change after their children were born, their wives did.

The following quote is from a 30-year-old woman who has been married to her 34-year-old husband for less than one year. She told us that they met online, fell in love, and she became pregnant two months later. They married two months after that. She went from sex goddess to untouchable mommy in less than twelve months.

> I had a baby seven weeks ago. Our sex life was fantastic, several times a day, before I became pregnant. For the last five months of pregnancy he said he couldn't make love to me because I was pregnant, but assured me that after the baby was born he would want me so much that I would get tired of him. Now that the baby is here he uses that as an excuse, but he won't talk about it. I'm the one who asks for sex and he says "no," or "maybe later." He even says "yes, but later." But later never comes. We used to be so sexual. Now nothing. I feel he isn't attracted to me anymore. And it is the most painful thing ever. I want my prepregnancy husband back.

Her husband probably wants his prepregnancy wife back, too. He may be terrified of all his new responsibilities—a carefree young guy one year, husband and father the next, with no period of adjustment. Not having any more sex may be insurance against not adding on additional responsibility. His wife doesn't think he's angry, just tired (no surprise there, with a new baby) and bored. But he could be quietly furious.

The following woman describes her husband's sexual interest as decreasing when she became his wife. Once she became the mother of his children, it was gone completely.

As soon as we married, even on the honeymoon, his sexual interest in me plummeted. Once we had kids, it was like he didn't need to have sex with me anymore. Either that was all he wanted from me, or I reminded him too much of "mother" and made him feel old. (Female, 51)

Some men spoke out about their feelings of suddenly realizing their wives were mothers. The following 34-year-old man describes it with clarity:

We had kids and by being in the labor room, I no longer saw my wife as the sexy woman that I married, but as a mother. Between my wife breast-feeding and the baby co-sleeping, it is hard to find the time, opportunity, or desire to have sex.

Whether a man admits it to himself or not, he might become jealous that he has a strong rival for his wife's love. Softly tender terms of endearment are now often directed at someone else. Or, in a variation of the previously mentioned Madonna/whore syndrome, the child's birth may confirm that his wife is no longer pure, and therefore undesirable. He may stop being a husband. Or he may be right. Dr. June Reinisch, director emerita of the Kinsey Institute, gives this caveat: "It's important for a woman to keep sexy. If she wants to have an erotic life with her partner, she does not want to turn herself into his mother."

Some men complained that *they* didn't change after their children were born, their wives did. A 59-year-old man, now divorced, wrote, "When she became a mother, she stopped being a wife." The following quote is from a 68-year-old man, married to a 67-year-old woman.

My wife says she has not enjoyed sex since the birth of her daughter forty years ago. She is not open to oral sex or any other options. I'm not interested in a younger body, only a partner who loves sex, is enthusiastic about it, is uninhibited, and loves to receive as well as give pleasure.

It is not uncommon for a woman to have a diminished sex drive after giving birth. This makes a good deal of biological sense; her immediate focus is on caring for the newborn. Fatigue, hormonal shifts, fear of discomfort or another pregnancy, and insecurity about her appearance may also be contributing factors. This is usually a temporary thing, lasting a few months to a year.

Occasionally a woman's sex drive never returns after having a baby. Forty years ago, the woman described in the preceding quote may have experienced a female variation of the Madonna/whore complex. Her child eclipsed her husband completely, leading to a shift that made physical intimacy inappropriate. She may have believed that sex was for procreation only, and once she became a mother, it was irrelevant, or even wrong.

five

PREDICTABLE, BORING, UNADVENTUROUS SEX

The message I get from sex is get it in, get it over with, and don't come back any time soon. **(Male, 60, married to his 60-year-old wife for forty-one years)**

When a sociologist interviewed twenty-two hundred American women in the 1920s, 25 percent of them said that when they had their first sexual experience, it "repelled" them. Even if they came to enjoy married sex, they were embarrassed to admit it. It just wasn't the ladylike thing to do. Passion was something base, something to be hidden; if a woman felt aroused, it was her secret. A radical Vassar College professor instructed: "a woman may conscientiously allow herself to feel passion to the same extent as the man, if she controls its expression." In spite of female lust hidden under the covers, there were surely wives who thoroughly enjoyed making love with their husbands or, perhaps, their lovers. In another survey, 25 percent of American men *and* women admitted to having experienced at least one affair.

It was a Faustian bargain. Men had a lot of reasons to want women's sexuality suppressed, and women, in general, seemed willing to at least pretend to suppress it. A lusty female was a threat; she might stray or become impregnated by another man who wouldn't have to foot the child-rearing bill. She might demand more in bed, expect a partner with skill, or have experienced a more talented lover. She might even have had "a past." Far better to invent a world in which a wife endured rather than enjoyed sex, even if she wasn't all that exciting a bed partner. If a man could afford it, he had a mistress or visited prostitutes; either was preferable to masturbation, an act that many social, political, and religious reformers of the time considered one of the most heinous things a man could do. (That belief lingered on for a long time. "Self-abuse" was considered harmful until the fairly recent past; in the 1950s, both the American Medical Association and the Boy Scout Manual stated it was something to be avoided.)

Since having sex with "good girls" was out of the question and masturbation was considered hazardous to one's health, prostitutes became the middle-class man's sexual rite of passage. These were the women from whom he got his "experience" and how he became a man of the world. In 1918, Dr. Marie Stopes (daughter of the feminist Charlotte Stopes who was the first woman in Scotland to graduate from college) wrote a wonderfully radical book titled *Married Love: A New Contribution to the Solution of Sex Difficulties.* She had a hard time getting it published. It stated marriage should be an equal relationship between husband and wife, and birth control readily available to all who wanted it, and it contained perhaps the most radical theory of all—those "good girls" who became wives were not only capable of, but longed for, intense sexual pleasure; for a happy marriage, their husbands had to give it to them, and she would explain how. Stopes eventually found a small publisher in London, where the book went on to be a big success. (After it was a bestseller in England, it was published in America, where the courts quickly declared it obscene and it was banned.) In the following passage, Dr. Stopes warns male newlyweds about confusing bought-and-paid-for sex with real life. In other words, don't think that because your wife doesn't act like a hooker, she doesn't enjoy sex, something some men in this century seem to forget to remember when they watch pornography.

> Many men, who enter marriage sincerely and tenderly, may yet have some previous experience of bought "love." . . . They argue that, because the prostitute showed physical excitement and pleasure in the sexual act, if the bride or wife does not do so, then she is "cold" or "undersexed." They may not realize that often all the bodily movements of the prostitute are studied and simulated because her client enjoys his orgasm best when he imagines that the woman in his arms has one simultaneously.

Of course, women of the late nineteenth and early twentieth centuries were not oddly lacking in libido; the times just made it convenient for them to pretend to be. "Hysteria" (from the Greek word for womb) was a commonly diagnosed "disease," and those with money to pay for sex but nowhere to shop went to popular hydrotherapy centers for "the cure." There, strong blasts of water aimed below the waist gave relief. Doctors also frequently massaged a female patient's pelvic area to help alleviate hysteria—the mechanical vibrator was developed to enable a female to do this on her own.

A significant American feminist movement, focusing on women's rights (suffrage, dress reform, and free love), happened at this time. Free love, by the way, did not mean sexual freedom. It was the belief that a woman had the right to control her own body, and that desire, not law, should dictate a sexual encounter. In other words, a wife shouldn't have to submit to her husband's advances unless she wanted to. (Marie Stopes considered this to be, in no uncertain terms, rape.) Around this time, some of the early therapists and advice givers began to suggest that the extreme suppression of female sexuality encouraged during the Victorian era might not be a good thing for marital success. As early as 1912, sex educator William Robinson had argued: "Every case of divorce has for its basis lack of sexual satisfaction." A book wrapped in plain brown paper became available to the discreet who were looking for ways to spice up their private lives. *How I Kept My Husband,* an oral sex how-to guide for women, cost ten cents.

Over the next few decades a woman's right to sexual pleasure increased; marriage was now supposed to supply at least some gratification to both participants. In 1950s America, with divorce rates at an all-time high, men finally had to worry about how to keep their wives satisfied in bed. In 1971, a University of Connecticut academic paper examined the eighteen bestselling marriage manuals of 1950 to 1970, to identify changes in the perception of female sexuality. The authors concluded that the male was still considered to be the dominant and more experienced partner, although, at long last, "greater female initiative and 'cooperation' is advocated." In other words, women were permitted to reveal some, but not all, of their sexuality and passion. They suggest that a wife might be on safe ground saying she enjoyed dinner, as long as she doesn't ask for a second helping when they state: "Radical implications of research on the multiorgasmic potential of women are virtually ignored in these books." The following year, 1972, would see a radical change in marriage manuals with the publication of Alex Comfort's *The Joy of Sex,* which stayed on the *New York Times* bestseller list for seventy weeks. Women were, for the first time in the twentieth century, depicted as not only sexual beings, but sexual equals.

But even before *The Joy of Sex,* a married woman was no longer expected to lie back and think of England. She could fantasize about having sex with the entire Royal Navy as long as she had a ring on the third finger of her left hand. Finally, she had permission to have a great time in bed. And that meant her partner had to provide it, and she had to give something back in return. For the married men and women of the 1950s and 1960s, the heat was on.

Today, American women are perceived of as being sexually liberated. Beginning with another major feminist movement in the 1960s, and helped along by everything from birth control pills to morning after pills to erectile dysfunction pills (with the promise of libido-enhancement pills in the future), women, whether married or not, have earned the right to as much sexual pleasure as men. Some might even argue more. Unlike the penis, the clitoris is an organ designated for pleasure alone. Few men are multiorgasmic, and as we've openly known for decades, many women are. It was therefore surprising to us that "she is not sexually adventurous" was the main reason, by far, that our male respondents gave for not having sex with their wives. Almost 70 percent of the men said this was the case. In addition, 61 percent said that their partners "did not seem to enjoy sex."

> She doesn't want anything except same place, same time, same way, and that's always with the TV taking priority. (Male, 57, married to his 55-year-old wife for thirty-four years)

We are aware that "not adventurous" can mean many things, from saying no to an open marriage to saying no to a new position, from refusing to go to a swinger's club to refusing to leave the lights on, and from experimenting with S&M to experimenting with sexy lingerie. The majority of male respondents, however, did not seem to be looking for anything out of the mainstream, just a little positive reinforcement.

> When we have sex, she lies on her back motionless. She has been like this in the almost nineteen years I have known her. Communication with her is difficult with mundane things like "what do you want for dinner," so a sexual discussion would seem completely out of the question. A few years ago I asked her to do something different, and I seem to remember that her response was simply "I don't do that." (Male, 40s)

This man is angry about more than sexual disinterest; he feels personally rejected by his wife. Although she may, on rare occasions, "allow" him to have sex with her, she is still punishing him by refusing to react, or by doing anything to contribute to his pleasure. She is also making it quite clear that she really wants nothing to do with intimacy—it is just her ultimate sacrifice.

Although it's possible that his partner lacks a sense of adventure in the bedroom, he was probably aware of this when he married her. However, the relationship evolved over the years into one filled with bitterness and hate. Small grievances, left unchecked, grew large. In a follow-up interview, he describes a woman who is either screaming, or giving him the silent treatment. His response is to avoid any and all conflict, and see himself as the good, sane guy and his wife as the selfish, crazy lady. Clearly, she is filled with anger, although he doesn't try to explain why, and perhaps he has never asked her. He does mention that the decline in their sex life occurred in 1992—she refused to have sex with him for two years after their first child was conceived. It seems evident that she resents her career choice of housewife and mother: "If I tell her something good happened at work, she responds with something like: 'That's nice. I don't get to have a career because I'm too busy cleaning the house and taking care of the kids.'" Jealousy of his life outside the home seems to consume her, and feeling unappreciated, she has become a dissatisfied, stay-at-home martyr.

I'm game for almost anything, but her idea of adventurous sex is leaving the light on. (Male, 30s)

Unless religious or moral reasons preclude sex prior to marriage, most people are aware of their partner's level of experimentation long before they marry. In a follow-up interview, the man in the preceding quote wrote that everything was great in the first few years: "We would often tell each other 'I want your body' and sent coded pager messages that translated to the same." Then she wanted to have a baby but had trouble conceiving. Suddenly, like countless other women in the same situation, she was only interested in sex when she thought she was ovulating. She had several miscarriages. Finally she carried to term, and then the sex became sporadic, although they had two more children.

We asked him if he ever asked her why she lost interest in sex after the birth of their first child. He replied that she suffers from migraines, backache, bad knees, and scars from the childbirth. Less than sympathetic, he says, "She just turned 40 and the girl is a wreck." But clearly he is hurt and angry when he adds he would feel much better about being turned down if she ever said, "Gee, I don't feel good, but boy, if I did . . ."

However, he then says that she has regained interest in the past few months, but he is reluctant due to a fear of having more children! This couple is on a merry-go-round of rejection, and calling his wife unadventurous covers up far more serious issues.

My wife was raised in a strict religious home and cannot release her inhibitions. She refuses anything but the straight, man-on-top position. She considers it beneath her and sinful to be sensuous. (Male, 76, married to his 70-year-old wife for forty years)

The preceding is less a question of sexual adventure than sexual boredom, and after forty years of the same thing, it just doesn't seem worth the effort to the husband anymore. His wife's religious beliefs are too deeply ingrained for her to ever change.

The next quotation is from a man who says he is angry, depressed, and has difficulty reaching orgasm. He is 40, his wife is 41.

Sex is boring, monotonous, and predictable when it happens. It's so much easier to just masturbate and be done with it.

Since he suffers from inhibited ejaculation, he probably climaxes with less difficulty during solitary sex. When he says that masturbation is preferable, he means it. Sex has become tedious; he's looking to climax and get it over with.

WHAT DOES "SEXUALLY ADVENTUROUS" MEAN, ANYWAY?

Here's what a 53-year-old man, who has had infrequent sex with his 52-year-old wife for the past five years of their twenty-eight-year marriage, had to say when, in a follow-up interview, we asked what he meant when he "strongly agreed" that his wife lacked sexual adventure.

> After thirty otherwise blissful years together, she is generally obstinately against any variations in sexual positions, techniques, or locations.

What would he like her to do differently?

> Being a man and visually stimulated, I have asked that she dress up provocatively for me; for example, she could wear the nylons and garter belt I bought her. Leave the lights on, look me in the eye, be open to suggestion, initiate sex, and enjoy each other's body in every way until God takes it away.

What is her reaction to these suggestions?

> She says I have her in every other way, but feels intimidated because she is uncomfortable with her body.

Is this a man married to a Victorian woman who thinks being a good girl and a sexy one is mutually exclusive? Have their years really always been "blissful"? Although he doesn't say he's angry, he mentions that after his business failed following 9/11, he didn't earn any income for two years. During this period, "My wife punished me by withholding intimacy. She wouldn't even kiss me, which is my barometer." He also says that his perimenopausal wife suffers from vaginal dryness, multiple yeast infections, and depression. It is certainly possible that he is angry at his wife for withholding sex during his difficult two-year period of unemployment, stopped having sex with her in retaliation, and that her physical problems have substantially lowered her libido to a point where she is grateful for this. "Not sexually adventurous" could be a convenient cover-up for them both. As we said, it can mean a lot of different things, some of them having nothing at all to do with adventure or sex. For example, the following 35-year-old man explains it this way:

> When we make love she is just receiving. I am doing all the touching and massaging. She doesn't respond back and arouse me in the same way. She also needs a vibrator to get and stay aroused, which interferes with our lovemaking positions and can affect my concentration.

He is responding negatively to his 35-year-old wife's sex toys. He may even be threatened by them. They have been married for four years and have sex less than once a month. She is "adventurous" enough to use a vibrator and masturbate openly during coitus, but shows no enthusiasm for him. He also mentions that she has gained weight and is working overtime to help pay their bills. She may be feeling less attractive because of the extra pounds or she may just be tired. Nevertheless, he wants a cheerleader, but is barely getting his season ticket punched, and she wants someone sensitive to her needs, someone who can get and keep her as interested as her vibrator. His "touching and massaging" isn't doing it for her; she may, in fact, think him lacking in sexual talent. They both may be angry and boring in bed. Unfortunately, they aren't talking about it.

When we asked sex therapist Janice Epp what she thought men meant by "not sexually adventurous" she told us: "Sometimes a partner will make the accusation as a bludgeon to hurt the other for perceived past hurts. And sometimes it's true." If true, why would a man choose such a partner? Epp believes that some men have a sense of superiority if they feel that their wife is sexually unadventurous; it gives them a certain advantage. Conversely, they would be threatened if she were experimental.

In other words, he can be that dominant, "experienced" guy of the first half of the twentieth century, living in a world where satisfying his wife isn't all that important, while she keeps her vibrator hidden away from him in the bottom of her drawer, where it belongs.

Is "Not Sexually Adventurous" Code for "No Oral Sex"?

There was a scene on an episode of HBO's *Lucky Louie* when Louie and his wife, Kim, who are having marital problems, are advised by a member of the clergy to really talk to each other, to privately share all the anger and resentments that have been bottled up during their five-year marriage. Now it's Louie's turn: "Sometimes, when we're having intercourse, I fantasize that you're blowing me," he confesses, adding, after a few beats, "actually, all the time." It brings down the house.

One of the biggest predictors of male sexual satisfaction is receiving oral sex.

According to a recent Elle Magazine/MSNBC poll of approximately 39,000 men, one of the biggest predictors of male sexual satisfaction is receiving oral sex. However, 45 percent of the approximately 39,000 women surveyed said that they don't like performing fellatio. A man wanting oral sex but not getting it at home is an ancient problem—red lipstick originated as a way for prostitutes to advertise their willingness to fellate their customers. There seems to be a real dichotomy here. Psychiatrist, sex therapist, and author Avodah K. Offit wrote, "When one considers that a partner can administer to the entire male region—testicle, anus, and buttocks as well as the penis—with hands and mouth, the wonder seems to be that men like intercourse at all."

Men view fellatio as an ultimate expression of love, commitment, adoration, tenderness, and temporary surrender. Unlike intercourse, it's also a time for a guy to just sit back and enjoy the ride, which may be the easiest explanation for its wide appeal. But many women, because of anger, or because they were never asked, or because they simply don't enjoy doing it, are not willing to make this a part of their lovemaking. The following quotations are a few examples of numerous variations on the same theme:

Wife is not open to oral sex or other options. (Male, 68/ Wife, 67)

When we have sex (five times last year), I have to make the first move and then it is the straight missionary position. She is not adventurous, so no question of oral or other activities. (Male, 52/ Wife, 47)

She has one position and that's it, never changes. No foreplay. No oral sex. (Male, 60/ Wife, 49)

She always thought that oral sex was "dirty" and something "normal people" just did not do. The few times we tried, it was obvious that she felt pressured to do it. (Male, 42)

But are these men performing cunnilingus if their wives want them to? In the Elle Magazine/MSNBC survey we mentioned earlier,

58 percent of the men claimed that their partner doesn't like receiving oral sex, although only 20 percent of the women said they were uncomfortable with the act.

We are not suggesting that any person should do something he or she is uncomfortable with, but we will unequivocally state that not giving is a sure way of not receiving.

> Most times, she was fairly disengaged, and wanted to get it over with as quickly as possible. She would sometimes "allow" me to perform oral sex on her, and that was one of the few ways I was able to get her involved. She would not reciprocate. (Male, 40s)

It is possible that men who claim their wives aren't sexually adventurous aren't particularly adventurous themselves. If, however, a woman won't perform fellatio, and her husband really wants her to and he is willing to lustily give her oral sex in return, we would urge her to rethink her position. Not giving oral sex can be a symbol of rejection to many men. And doing it can be a beautiful, healing, and, yes, sexy, thing. It can deepen a relationship, and be empowering—the giver is in control. It is also a wonderful thing to give pleasure to someone you love. If a woman is unsure of exactly what to do, there are a number of good books, but probably none better than any edition of *The Joy of Sex*. Unfortunately, *How I Kept My Husband* is no longer in print.

Is "Not Sexually Adventurous" Code for "She Isn't Giving Me Positive Feedback"?

If 68 percent of the men said their partners lacked adventure, almost as many said that their partners didn't seem to enjoy sex. This may be true, for a variety of reasons. He may not be doing anything all that enjoyable, or she may not be able to verbalize her feelings. For a lot of men, a partner who tells them they are sexy, hot, and terrific in bed becomes a great lover himself. That's pretty much all it takes. These guys don't want a silent partner, they want applause. Men tend to be goal oriented; they like to know that objectives have been reached.

Other men may be right; their wives may not have a lot of interest. These guys may be good lovers, or trying their best to be, but negative body image, health, anger, vaginal dryness, low libido, or a variety of other psychological or physiological issues may stop their wives from wanting or enjoying sex. Hurt, rejected, and not talking about it—they shut down.

> The emotional drain of having to ask for sex repeatedly, be promised, and then turned down became insulting. Being tossed a "favor" now and then is worse than having to buy sex, which I've never done. It is not the simple act of orgasm—that's easy enough to fix—but the idea of being wanted, touched, and satisfying someone else that is the real glue in a relationship. (Male, 30s)

Women frequently complain that they want more out of sex than just the end result; the man just quoted feels the same way. He wants an emotional connection; he wants to be loved. He thinks his wife is a tease, and that she sees lovemaking as a chore to be doled out in small amounts, because she has to.

> My wife likes cuddling but she doesn't like it when I try to be intimate. She will submit occasionally but then complain about how messy she feels. She seems to think that sex isn't for people over 50, and that I am obsessed by it. I never thought I would consider an affair, but I am considering one now. (Male, 54/ Wife, 51)

The couple in the preceding quote is on opposite sides of the bed. Her idea of intimacy and connecting is cuddling, his is sex. There is nothing wrong with either, but they are very different ways of expressing love. She is making him feel badly about wanting to have sex with his wife. He is withdrawing and fantasizing about an affair. Neither seem able to put themselves in their spouse's place, and sadly, they really aren't that far apart.

Is "Not Sexually Adventurous" Code for "She Doesn't Want Me Enough"?

Some of our male respondents complained that their wives were never the ones to suggest making love. In their minds, adventurous seems to mean any sign of enthusiasm, a seductive suggestion or touch, a feeling of being desired. The following quotations are from men who say they never feel desired.

> In my 40s, I decided to stop and wait for my wife to initiate some form of intimacy. It never happened, so I came to the conclusion she didn't like that part of me. My wife is still very attractive. I'm not sure why she lost her desire to stop being intimate. I guess I'm angry that I try to respect the things she likes and give her everything she wants, but my simple needs are not important to her. As you may be able to tell, we don't communicate very well but we have a very happy marriage otherwise. (Male, 57, married to his 59-year-old wife for thirty-five years)

This couple stopped having a sexual relationship ten years ago. At that time, the man decided to give his wife a test. He wasn't going to have sex with her unless she initiated. They had been married for twenty years or so and she was used to him being the aggressor. Since he didn't tell her the game had new rules, she likely thought *he* was no longer interested in making love to *her*. This might have caused her to be angry, or imagine an infidelity, or think that she was no longer attractive, especially since the rules changed right around the time she was beginning menopause. Who knows? She also may have been relieved. The point is, her husband never asked. He preferred to be angry, resentful, hurt, and celibate, stating the obvious when he says, "We don't communicate very well."

This man is trying hard to show what a great husband he is. He gives his wife "everything she wants" and is part of a "very happy marriage" in spite of the lack of sex and conversation. Although he may have set out to prove his wife really desired him, it's equally possible that he always knew she would fail the test. That way, he could stop having sex with her, and take no responsibility. The blame shifts to her; and he can believe she never really liked sex. In his mind, he's still the good guy.

> She doesn't have the interest, especially any adventuresome approach. She rarely makes the first move and often pushed me away. (Male, 54/ Wife, 51)

Many women still operate under the quaint rule that it's up to the man to initiate sex. But they don't say this, and the guy ends up feeling rejected. In the preceding case, however, her frequent rejection is compounding the problem. This man has given up. Whether or not he's doing anything to encourage passion isn't the point (he thinks he is); he's been turned down or put off so many times, sex no longer seems worth the effort.

> She has NEVER initiated sex, not once, in our married life together. (Male, 67, married for twenty-seven years)

One of the most popular male sexual fantasies is a sexually aggressive woman. She initiates, takes charge in bed, and tells him what to do and when to do it. It is the opposite of the role most men find themselves in. That being said, some of those same men may feel threatened if their partners suddenly became aggressive. Fantasies often don't play out very well when they become real.

WHO'S ON TOP?

For some men, the idea of a woman not being sexually adventurous enough may be code for control—specifically, who's in charge here? The 56-year-old man in the following quote complained that his wife called all the shots in bed:

> She controls the speed that I perform, the proper angles, how long it takes, and what positions we are in. Only the missionary will do. I long ago lost interest in her.

And this man in his 40s is married to a woman who plays the role of "expert," pointing out all the things that go wrong in bed:

> She became frequently critical of the affection I showed sexual or otherwise. Everything was too soon, too late, too much or too little. I eventually filtered the commentary out but in the process I lost interest in her on many levels. (Male, 40s)

The following 30-year-old man also indicates that his wife is a tough critic:

> When we were first married she led me to believe that she was somewhat naïve about sex. But she always seemed to find some little problem with our lovemaking, like not lasting long enough, not enough foreplay, or I was too quiet (I don't talk to her).

It is likely that this man wasn't very sexually sophisticated when he married, and it was less threatening that his wife seemed lacking in experience, too. Whether or not she was really sexually "naïve" is unimportant (and his hint that she wasn't indicates a serious lack of trust); her complaints about not enough foreplay and not lasting long enough are not "little problems" at all. They are serious issues and are preventing her from optimal enjoyment.

Most men are relieved to be told what their
wives want in bed.

She is communicating her needs, but without sensitivity. Hurt and angry, her partner isn't listening. And that's too bad. Most men are relieved to be told what their wives want in bed; a road map to keep them heading in the right direction can be very welcome. If this woman said something like "Sweetie, I really enjoy making love with you, but I need a little more time to get aroused. It would be wonderful if . . ." it would work a lot better than being critical. It is difficult to overemphasize how lacking in confidence most people are about their lovemaking skills.

NO SENSE OF ADVENTURE? SAYS WHO?

When asked if "I'm not sexually adventurous enough for him" was an accurate description of why their husbands stopped being intimate, the majority of our female respondents all but jumped up and shouted "Hell, no!" Eighty-six percent disagreed with this statement, and even more women (90%) disagreed with "I don't seem to enjoy sex." When asked "How sexual do you feel at this point in your life?" 56 percent said "intensely," or "very." Of those remaining,

27 percent considered themselves to be average. Less than 3 percent reported not feeling sexy at all. Many women seemed to think it was their husbands who are lacking in adventure, and more. A 35-year-old woman told us something reminiscent of so many of the male respondents: "He thinks oral sex and sex in any position other than missionary is perverted." A 45-year-old woman described her selfish and emotionally disconnected husband like this: "He tends to forget I'm there; he only worries about what he wants. He doesn't touch me very often, but always expects oral from me."

A 45-year-old registered nurse wrote that she was relieved that her physician husband stopped being sexual with her.

> He's a medical doctor so you would think he would have an edge with his extensive knowledge of anatomy and physiology. He doesn't have a clue. He is very clumsy, he usually turns all of the lights off, and he doesn't seem to know where his arms and legs are in relation to mine. Because of this he often pokes me. I tried candles so he could see. He would not bathe before sex and had body odor. When I realized he did not consider me special enough to want to please me I made a 360-degree turn and started to focus on myself. I finally told him to sleep in another bedroom and that if we are EVER sexual again it will be me who decides when it will occur and that our intimate relationship will have to be based on real attachment and not mindless sex. I am taking control of my own sexuality.

We asked her what that meant.

> I love erotica (romance stories). I still believe in love. I do not have a problem with sex toys. Right now I am learning what I like and what is good for me. I am not trying to please someone else. I refuse to participate in bad sex. I want quality, meaningful sex. Otherwise, he can keep it.

We also asked what she thought the future would be for them as a couple.

> He is very motivated. He has gone to our pastor and admitted he has been selfish and unloving. He is going into counseling and allowing himself to be mentored by other men in the church. When he makes some progress, I will join him in counseling. We are finally talking, and he is open to learning how to be a "good lover." He is examining his insecurities about sex. I am trying to get him to understand that marriage is supposed to be a safe place. If he can learn these things, there is hope.

Sex in a long-term marriage will probably never be as frequent and delicious as it once was, and if that's what you expect, you are setting yourself and your partner up to fail.

In an earlier chapter, we spoke of the need for individualization and creativity to keep a marriage sexually active. The woman we just quoted who has decided to start taking responsibility for her own happiness may well discover that when her husband realizes she isn't someone to take for granted and is more like a new pair of spike heels than an old pair of sneakers, her marriage improves dramatically.

We'll say it again: sex in a long-term marriage will probably never be as frequent and delicious as it once was, and if that's what you expect, you are setting yourself and your partner up to fail. But that doesn't mean it can't be good, and a regular part of your life.

One respondent said his wife wasn't sexually adventurous because she refused to enter into a polyamorous (accepted multiple partners) relationship, and another talked about "swinging." Although some may fantasize about these types of arrangements, few couples make it a reality, because frankly, this isn't for most people. While it may be true that shaking up a relationship's foundation reignites a few sparks, we think it's more likely to burn down the house. It is beyond dispute that a new partner might be exciting, and extramarital relations revealed may actually activate some hormones and temporarily restore passion. However, we live in a culture strongly based on fidelity. Jealousy is a volatile emotion, and even if it jump-starts lust, it stands a good chance of destroying love.

six

ANGER MISMANAGEMENT

Some people seem to be living in a marriage that's like an onion—they peel away one piece of resentment after another, until there is only an empty core. Nothing does a better job of killing intimacy than layers of built-up rage; it was therefore not surprising that so many of our respondents were mad as hell. Forty-four percent of the men said, "I am angry at her," and 45 percent of the women agreed that their husbands were furious. When asked why, the men claimed anger was a justifiable reaction to their partner's negative behavior. The word *critical* appeared regularly, an important ingredient in the formula for sexual Novocain.

Nothing does a better job of killing intimacy
than built-up rage.

She is frequently critical of any affection I show, sexual or otherwise. Everything is too much, too little, too soon, too late. I eventually learned to filter the negative commentary, but in the process I lost interest in her on many levels. **(Male, 50s)**

Although this man complains that his wife is critical, he also writes that he used to work an incredible eighty to one hundred hours every week. His wife called his work habits "insulting," especially since he was often too tired to be intimate. They each seem well practiced in figuring out how to offend the other, and the resulting absence of passion may actually be preferable to them both.

> She is critical of everything I do. Examples include my appearance, the way I dress, my friends, how I drive, the way I eat, my choice of everything from restaurants to parking spaces. (Male, 60s)

There is no greater gift in life than the joy one gets from passion born out of love, and no better way to destroy it than the inability to deal with anger correctly. It is no surprise that the preceding man has stopped being sexual; his performance would probably be just one more item on his partner's list of what he does to annoy her.

> I realize that sex with her gave her the power to hurt me, as she was verbally and mentally abusive. I broke off all contact with her. (Male, 40s)

It has been theorized that the absence of sexual desire is most often related to expressed or unexpressed anger. Many men who responded to our survey said they were angry at their wives because their wives were always angry at them. They were living with critical and controlling women who were ready to fly off the handle for any reason at all; the only thing missing from their descriptions were pointy black hats and brooms. We don't believe anger is one-sided, or, at least, it rarely is, but a lot of respondents seem to perceive of it that way. They are taking no responsibility for, or are oblivious to, their part in the story.

She is always in a bad mood, putting me down and showing her displeasure with her life and me. (Male, 40)

A conflict-free relationship is impossible. However, when conflict becomes either a cause or an excuse for withholding sex, it is not being handled properly.

Sex therapists Gerald Weeks and Nancy Gambescia mention a variety of ways couples deal with anger that they consider "incompatible with sexual desire." Some people don't censor; they say hurtful and inappropriate things without considering the impact. Others are constantly angry, ready to explode for any reason at all. In both of these cases, the "nonangry" partner lives in constant terror that something (*anything*) they say might set off an explosion.

One female respondent, now divorced, described marriage to her raging ex-husband this way:

I stayed way too long! The funniest and saddest day was when we attempted joint therapy. The counselor had to ask him to keep his voice down and to stop yelling at her and me. The sad thing is that my ex is brilliant and has a Ph.D. in the field of languages. It seemed absurd that he acted that way. The therapist was so scared she called the security guard! (Female, 57)

ANGER CAN DESTROY PASSION, AND USUALLY DOES

It is unlikely that anyone would want to make love to a screaming bully of a spouse. Uncontrollable rage can be a sign of chemical imbalance, a result of alcohol or drug abuse, self-loathing, or just an effective method of avoiding sex and intimacy. If the more tranquil partner has a fear of intimacy and commitment as well, he or she may have found an excellent way of avoiding sex without taking any of the responsibility. It is also possible that the calm spouse is so afraid of being left alone, or feels so unworthy of a loving relationship, that he or she is willing to choose a bad marriage over none. Those who grew up in a household with an abusive or alcoholic parent sometimes replicate their childhood environment in marriage, choosing a mate who is disagreeable but comfortable—the devil they know. The marriage may seem no worse, or even a bit better than what they experienced as children, and therefore acceptable.

Men frequently use anger to cover up sexual anxiety.

But if a woman still desires intimacy with her raging spouse, possibly confusing fury with passion, the angry partner has effectively created a platform of refusal. Men frequently use anger to cover up sexual anxiety. As unpleasant as an argument may be, it's preferable to facing the humiliation of unaddressed sexual dysfunction. Not getting or sustaining an erection can also be a way of passively showing contempt. Withholding sex becomes a punishment; he is refusing to give her something she wants, perhaps one of the few things he perceives as still being within his control. For example, a 60-year-old man, married to his 50-year-old wife for five years, wrote that he cut off all sexual relations in the second year of marriage because "she tells me what I'm doing wrong all the time." However, he also mentions that he suffers from ED but has not seen a doctor and chooses to watch pornography online for twenty-eight hours a week. He is classically covering up his impotence while taking back the little control he has over his sex life by getting solitary relief without fear of humiliation. The anger that he is feeling toward himself, fueled by his wife's criticism, may destroy the marriage unless both decide to confront these serious issues. It is even possible that his anger is the cause of his impotence.

THE ULTIMATE INTIMACY KILLER

For the constantly critical, anger is often a first line of defense against intimacy and commitment. The foundation may be a deeply serious wound, like a discovered or confessed infidelity, or an assortment of trivial complaints that seem, on the surface, to be meaningless.

> I think I'm too critical of him sometimes. I have high standards for how a person should be. I am critical of the way he walks around the house. He walks on his heels instead of the balls of his feet. That makes the whole house shake. (Female, 30s)

The "noncritical" or "nonangry" partner responds by withholding touch, warmth, and sex, which gives the "angry" spouse more reason to stay that way. Both are certain their choice is valid. What man would want to get close to a woman who despises him? What woman wouldn't feel justified being angry at a man who refuses to touch her?

Although one plays the role of the openly angry spouse, it can be in response to a partner who is either quietly hostile, or so emotionally shut down that his or her frustration and attempt at control is inevitable. One partner may also be passive-aggressive, seemingly compliant and loving, but not. This can show up in a variety of ways, by "forgetting" to do things that were promised, or by consistently being late. If he thinks of his wife as an authority figure, this can be a convenient way of retaliating without taking any risk. It will probably result in criticism, but that further justifies his silent anger. As one 63-year-old woman who has been married for forty-four years wrote:

He is passive-aggressive. He doesn't yell or argue a lot, but will NOT do anything I suggest, either in bed or around the house.

Of course, men can be the constantly critical partner, too:

He is very critical in general, always complaining, but really he doesn't want to have sex. For example, he won't have sex if the clothes aren't all put away, or if a TV show he likes is on. There isn't any consistency; he makes up excuses as he goes along. (Female, 37)

This man is pretending to use sex for both punishment and reward, but it's all an illusion. She's right in thinking his manipulative behavior is masking the fact that he really doesn't want sex. From his perspective, *she* has become the reason for his lack of desire—if the laundry were just put away properly, he would want to make love.

And sometimes, they are equals in critical warfare:

We are often angry with each other. She is quick to criticize or at least bicker and I'm quick to be defensive. (Male, 59)

Cohabitation or marriage does not guarantee closeness, and if one or both partners fear intimacy, anger and resentment can be effectively used to prevent it. In addition, anger can be reassuring—if the relationship ends, the loss might be bearable. In other words, not being fully committed to the marriage is an insurance policy against future vulnerability. (The converse, never fighting, has the same result. Both partners are so emotionally codependent that for either to exert control and express anger is impossible because it would mean taking responsibility for what might go wrong. Arguing could lead to abandonment. Unfortunately, when all conflict is eliminated, passion usually is, too.)

HE MAY JUST BE ANGRY AT HIMSELF

Constant criticism may also mask insecurity. If a man feels unsuccessful or inadequate, why would anyone love him or want to make love to him? If his partner still desires him, there must be something wrong with her. When (and if) he tries to talk about his problems, his partner may be so emotionally battered that she has stopped listening. Eventually, as a kind of Pygmalion myth in reverse, he may transmogrify the woman he loves into the angry, disappointed, and bitter partner he thinks he deserves.

> He is very angry at me, because I am successful in my career, and he isn't. He treats me with disdain, saying I am a terrible mother and a "hostile bitch." Maybe he's right, now I'm angry all the time, too. (Female, 30)

This woman's husband is taking no responsibility for his own life, choosing instead to pretend all of his problems originate with the woman he married. He has turned her into what he thinks he ought to have—a woman angry at him for his lack of success.

> I am not sure why he is so angry at me; I just know that he is. I guess he blames me for everything in his life that didn't turn out the way he hoped it would. (Female, 49)

This woman sees herself as a scapegoat. In a follow-up interview, she writes that her husband watches pornography on a regular basis, has had an affair, and suffers from ED without seeking a cure, so it is difficult to imagine that she isn't angry at him, too. She describes herself as having gained a significant amount of weight; perhaps this is a way for her to passively express it. This couple is using anger and accusation to disguise their extremely serious marital issues.

Instead of confronting those problems, they choose to be constantly enraged.

> He tells me he has nightmares about me dying. He described one to me—people were carrying a body bag and I was inside. He has made poor financial decisions and gone through a lot of my money. I have been very angry about that. We live in my house. (I bought it before I met him.) I feel he wants to share in my things, but resents it if he has to share anything with me. (Female, 56)

This woman also writes that she has recently changed from a slim, health-conscious jogger to an overweight person with multiple medications and hypertension. Her husband is nine years younger than she and seems to be terribly frightened that he will lose her to death, or that she will ask him to leave. However, they are also both very possessive and withholding people. After ten years of marriage, she still refers to the place they live in as "my house" and his bad investments as having been made with "my money," and he seems to believe that what belongs to his wife belongs to them both, but what belongs to him is his alone. He won't even share intimacy.

The following quote shows a 38-year-old man still angry about something that happened more than twenty years ago:

> She was promiscuous in high school; I was a "good" kid. Every year I resent our pasts more.

He has been holding on to this trump card for a generation. He married her fully aware that she was more sexually experienced than he was, but he can't stop judging her for what he considers to be prior indiscretions. He seems to be masking fear of inadequacy with his resentment about something that can never change.

SILENTLY SEETHING

Anger can also be a quiet thing, an emotion buried deep inside someone fearful that speaking up will be catastrophic. Gerald Weeks and
Nancy Gambescia say that in their experience, withholding anger is
the most common pattern of all, and men are somewhat more likely to
do it than women. "The internalized anger becomes a chronic condition that we call *chronically suppressed anger.* These partners are filled
with bitterness and smoldering resentment. . . . Suppressed anger becomes the pervasive state and blocks the experience of all other feelings, including sexual desire. These individuals often appear pensive,
depressed, anxious, or withdrawn. They are likely to remain emotionally disengaged from their partners in order to remain quietly angry."

*The only way to try to eliminate hostility is to talk
about the issues.*

Dr. Robert Mendelsohn, a psychoanalyst and couple's therapist on
Long Island, New York, who believes that the number one reason men
stop being sexual with their wives is anger, told us that often men
present a long list of unexpressed resentments. They remain unspoken
because the man would rather withdraw from conflict than deal with
it. He calls this "pathologically polite"—angry but refusing to say so
out of fear that once one set of grievances is out in the open, his partner may counterattack with a set of her own. (However, he says some
male patients do complain openly, especially about their spouse's criticism. He has noticed a shift in his patients over the past ten to fifteen
years, with men complaining their wives are "whiney and nagging"
and women complaining about not getting enough sex.) Clinical sex-
ologist Janice Epp believes that men are frequently unable to express

anger: "Very often, men enter a relationship with virtually no communication skills. Women are socialized to be communicators and nurturers, so when the inevitable conflicts arise, women want to process
and discuss. Many men report they feel backed into a corner. They
bury their anger and shut down."

The only way to try to eliminate hostility is to talk about the issues.
There simply is no other way. The choices become easier if you consider the options: either confront some painful, uncomfortable things,
or continue being unhappy until the marriage disintegrates. It's important to communicate in a way the other person can understand. Let's
consider a common problem—a woman is angry that most of the burden
of housework falls on her. If she starts with negativity, all her spouse
will hear are those first derogatory words. For example, if the conversation begins with "You're lazy," that's all her husband will hear, even
though she may go on to logically explain why she feels justified in
making the statement. What she should do is express her grievances,
and then suggest a solution. For example: "I think the house is messy.
I know that this bothers me more than it does you, and maybe it's because most of the responsibility to clean and do laundry seems to be
left up to me. We both work hard, and housework isn't any fun. But
maybe if we work together for an hour every day, the house will look a
lot better, and it would be a lot easier on me." We are aware that having this type of conversation is unpleasant, and that silence may seem
preferable. It's so much easier to go for a solitary walk or to turn on the
television. If the issues are more serious, or one or both partners have
difficulty communicating, a therapist or member of the clergy might
be of benefit. And sometimes outside help can be a bit more problem
specific; for example, hire a maid, or send out the laundry if you can
afford to do so. (In the case of our imaginary couple, it would be
worthwhile to cut back on *anything* to be able to do this. Do they really
need another premium cable channel?) But we can't say this enough—
you won't solve anything unless you talk to each other, in a way you
can both understand. And listen.

WHAT IF HE WON'T TALK?

The problem about talking is this—often men refuse to do it, particularly when the topic is something that threatens their masculinity. And, as we mentioned, both men and women can lack the vocabulary and communication skills necessary to talk about sexual starvation. The following comment is from a 51-year-old woman married for thirty-one years. Her husband, also 51, suffers from erectile dysfunction and rapid ejaculation, and he has difficulty achieving orgasm. He stopped all sexual contact, including hugging and kissing, six years ago.

> He claims he has no interest in sex and since he doesn't, I shouldn't, either. He says I should just learn to live with it. It is not a topic he will discuss in any way, shape, or form. Discussion on this topic is forbidden. (Female, 51)

She requested that her husband go into therapy with her, but he refused. (Forty-four percent of our female respondents said they wanted their husbands to go into couple's therapy, but were turned down.) We asked Dr. Reinisch how a woman should handle a situation like this, where a husband adamantly refuses therapy and the marriage may end if they don't get help. She suggests approaching the situation as the mutual problem it is, saying something like: "Sweetie, I understand you're reluctant to do something about this, but this marriage means so much to me, our relationship and communication on every level means so much. Sexuality means so much to me. I know this problem is ours, so I'm going to take care of my half, I'm going into therapy. You can join me if and when you're ready."

Dr. Reinisch believes this almost always works, because "It is a very rare man who can stand the fact that his wife has gone off to couple's therapy without him." Why is this? What is he afraid of?

"That she's talking about him! And she's telling both her side and his side."

Sometimes it's the woman who refuses therapy. Twenty-five percent of the men who responded to our survey said so. This 51-year-old male has been married to his 51-year-old wife for thirty-two years: "I am angry at her. She wants to control everything and run the whole marriage. Everything *has* to be done how she wants, when she wants, and she absolutely refuses to discuss sex." He told us that he asked her repeatedly to go into therapy with him, but she wouldn't. So he is in therapy alone, and, he says, thinking about having an affair.

JUSTIFIABLE ANGER

There are the small annoyances that get discussed rationally and forgotten quickly in a well-functioning relationship, and then there is deeply justifiable anger. One example of this is the hell of living with an alcoholic or drug-abusive partner who is unwilling to change.

A recently divorced but still furious 50-year-old man says about his 48-year-old ex-wife: "My anger is related to her alcoholism. She fell off the wagon and usually passed out by 8 P.M."

Long-term alcoholism causes ED, lowers testosterone production, and destroys testicular cells.

A 51-year-old woman married to a 51-year-old alcoholic for twenty-six years said her husband stopped having sex with her nine years ago. Frustrated and angry, she has a litany of resentments that goes back decades: "He was disinterested in planning the wedding. He told me 'I'm not a babysitter' when I asked him to help out with our first-born." She says that she is seriously considering divorce, but is unsure of when because of her children. She has also had an affair. She believes her husband is very angry at her

> . . . because I have pointed out the alcoholic problems, gone to Al-Anon, have conducted an intervention, told him that I don't like that he gambles and watches online porn, and that I have forced him to attend counseling. He is angry because I no longer tolerate his verbal abuse.

She also says that her husband "views sex as recreational and cannot understand the need for emotional attachment first." His pornography "addiction" might be due to impotence, a natural by-product of alcoholism. Large quantities of alcohol prevent erections, and long-term alcoholism causes ED, lowers testosterone production, and destroys testicular cells. Every female survey respondent who mentioned alcoholism also said that her husband suffered from ED.

WITHHOLDING SEX AS PUNISHMENT

Often adults re-create what they learned as children; for example, bad behavior means no dessert. This can result in sex, ideally a loving and pleasurable way to connect with one's partner, becoming just another commodity to be traded for actions deemed commendable. If she's a good girl, she may get two helpings, but if she's bad, like a child sent to the "time-out" room for misbehaving, it's off to bed without your sex!

> I often find myself holding back sexually because I'm too busy remembering ten years of being hurt and rejected and can't move past it. (Male, 50s)

Infidelity, of course, is the ultimate example of justifiable rage; betrayal produces anger that is understandable and valid. It threatens the core of the partnership, and if the reason for the infidelity is buried, and the conflict is neither explored nor resolved, the bitterness may last a lifetime. The wounded remain married, and they remain enraged, punishing their partners until death do them part.

This 68-year-old male respondent has been married to his 70-year-old wife for forty-eight years, but stopped having sex with her twenty-three years ago after he caught her in an affair: "We have stayed married but I will have nothing to do with her physically. I am still livid with her." He says that they plan to "live out our remaining years together," and when we asked him if he could do anything differently, what it would be, he replied: "Nothing. She made her bed, so now she has to lie in it." Rage is fueling his self-righteousness. Staying with her allows him to play the role he has become comfortable with, that of a victimized martyr.

And this 68-year-old man has been married to his 66-year-old spouse for forty years. In 1978, she found out that he was having an affair ("I possibly was a sex addict," he says). This discovery of infidelity was initially positive because the crisis forced him to get help, he promised to be faithful, and the intimate part of their marriage resumed. But then:

> All sexual conduct ceased in April 1984. We made love in the morning. That was the last time we were sexually active. She was 44 years old and I was 47. We do not sleep together. She sleeps in the second-floor bedroom, I in the first-floor family room. In hotels we ask for two queen beds. We both love each other; we just do not have sex and have not for twenty-two years.

When we inquired about the future, he replied that they intended to stay together forever and would hopefully die concurrently in their sleep many years from now. Just not in the same bed.

Others cannot survive infidelity. A male (60) and his wife (48) divorced because: "She cheated on me more than once, and I lost the desire to have sex with her." However, he also mentions that he suffers from erectile dysfunction, and "I felt I wasn't man enough for her anymore due to the fact she cheated." He's blaming himself twice—for his wife's infidelity and for his own impotence. She is currently married to the man with whom she had the affair.

It is not unusual for a crisis to temporarily result in restored passion.

And some couples not only survive infidelity, they emerge stronger. It has recently been theorized that when women become very comfortable in a marriage, and feel that there is no chance that their husband might stray, their libidos drop. Of course, the security of love and fidelity is one of the things that make marriage wonderful, but perhaps too much complacency inadvertently signals disinterest. The following 67-year-old woman loved her 75-year-old husband, but sex was infrequent for three years prior to September 11, 2001, when she discovered he was having an affair. She told us:

> My husband is the last man on earth that I thought would have an affair besides my dad and maybe Billy Graham. It began online and went on for twenty-one months until 9/11/2001, the day I found out. It actually brought us closer together, and we had the best sex of our entire marriage in 2002–2003, even at our ages. We worked through the problems, but now because of health issues we have lapsed back into the not-too-often routine. *[She said they made love ten times in the past year.]* We do hug and kiss a lot throughout the day. I think we will find

happiness from now on regardless of how often we make love; we will be together until death do us part.

In answer to the question "If you could do things over again, what would you do differently?" she replied, "Try to appreciate him more and let him know it."

It is not unusual for a crisis to temporarily result in restored passion. This woman discovered her husband was unfaithful on the most frightening and emotional day in recent American history, and their marriage and the world spun simultaneously out of control. One result of their personal trauma was renewed desire. They both feared losing the other so much that the respondent describes the type of intense passion that generally only appears during the first few months of a new and potentially long-term committed relationship, when brain chemicals might inspire a pair to bond as often as possible in order to facilitate attachment. This probably helped them heal, and also indicates the love they had for each other, despite what happened. This couple also appears to have approached the serious issues of their marriage with maturity and compassion. Realizing all they had to lose, they turned a catastrophe into an opportunity for a better, more loving, and stronger commitment. Instead of living out their lives filled with bitterness and resentment, they are sharing a renewed sense of love and mutual respect.

TODAY ANGER, TOMORROW APATHY

Say this about anger, at least it shows feeling and emotion. But sometimes, people metaphorically throw up their hands and choose not to feel angry. In fact, they choose not to feel anything.

I remember looking at her and realizing that I was no longer attracted to her. It was over. This also took away her last and most powerful manipulative tool and, yes, that made her even also identified as masturbating. Twenty-four percent were having affairs. Some were doing both. Men may use masturbation as a quick fix for depression. It can be an instant (if short-lived) mood enhancer. If anxiety accompanies depression, and it often does, masturbation may also be a temporary tranquilizer. So may a brief encounter. The guilt and fear that usually go along with an affair may be the cause of the depression; or the sexual relief possible in a nonintimate relationship may be purely analgesic.

WHAT CAUSES DEPRESSION?

Depression is believed to be the result of a chemical imbalance in the brain, but there is not yet a way to pinpoint the exact chemicals. Research suggests that it is likely one or more of the neurotransmitters serotonin, dopamine, or norepinephrine.

An estimated 19 million Americans suffer from depression. Needless to say, stress and trauma can lead to situational despair. Often, the healing powers of time or a change in the situation can sweep the depression away. But it is also possible that time does not heal all wounds, or that there was no "obvious" reason to begin with. It has been theorized that the body's inability to properly utilize nutrients may be a cause, and that genetic predetermination may be one as well. (Although a depression gene has yet to be identified, researchers believe there may be several.)

Clinically depressed people can't just "pull themselves together," anymore than people suffering from excruciating physical pain can just wish it away.

Women are statistically twice as likely to be depressed as men; however, this may be underestimated because men are less likely to seek psychiatric or medical help, which may be why men are four times more likely to commit suicide. Men are also more likely to try and mask their pain with anger, irritability, and alcohol abuse. This is

angrier. We continued to live in a sexless marriage for two years after that. It wasn't the first time we had gone for a long time without sex; at another point in our marriage she cut me off for sixteen months, but this time it was my decision. Sex was a weapon. We are divorced now, surprise, surprise. I don't miss her. And my dog is a heck of a lot more affectionate then she ever was. (Male, 50s)

This couple took turns using sex as a weapon until there was nothing left to fight for. Indifference empowered him, or, at least, he believed it did. She may have seemed angry, at first, that he no longer desired her, in spite of the fact that she had previously punished him in precisely the same way. In the final two years of the marriage, it is possible her hostilities diminished as well, and she became as apathetic as her husband. They didn't have anything to shake things up, certainly not open and honest conversation, and probably got to a point where neither could remember why they ever fell in love.

seven

DEPRESSION: THE ULTIMATE PASSION KILLER

I think that he may not have ever been very interested in sex. The signs were even there before we got married, but I ignored them. Then depression kicked in. He was no longer able to fake it and didn't even try to anymore. He never initiated and turned me down at least half the time I initiated. **(Female, 40, married for ten years)**

A person suffering from depression sees the world through gray-colored glasses. He is filled with negativity about the past, present, and future. The American Psychiatric Association's *Diagnostic and Statistical Manual* lists nine symptoms, which include:

- Feeling depressed most of the day nearly every day
- Markedly diminished pleasure
- Significant weight change
- Insomnia
- Agitation
- Fatigue and loss of energy
- Feelings of worthlessness and/or inappropriate guilt

- Diminished concentration
- Thoughts of suicide

It goes without saying that intimate, joyful, and passionate love-making is likely to be low on a depressed person's to-do list. Indeed, the effect of depression on libido has been described as devastating; it has been estimated that 70 percent of depressed people also suffer from a loss of desire. Some therapists claim a clinically depressed patient who retained desire would be a rarity.

---

70 percent of depressed people also suffer from a loss of desire.

Fifty-seven percent of our female respondents agreed that their husbands were depressed, and it was the main reason they believed their spouses were lacking sexual desire. (The majority of these women also said their partners were angry.) Of the male respondents, only 34 percent said they felt depressed, although like erectile dysfunction and premature ejaculation, this may be underreported. Thirty-six percent of the women said they themselves suffered from depression, and 40 percent of the men said that their wives were depressed.

The majority of the men who self-identified as depressed said their wives were depressed, too. It's possible that the wives were depressed because the husbands were. Or it could be, as the late psychologist George Bach observed, that water seeks its own level, and depressed people seek out depressed partners.

THE PARADOX OF SEX AND DEPRESSION

Can depression and sexual activity coexist? Sometimes they can. In our survey, half of the men who strongly agreed they were depressed likely why almost every female respondent who claimed her husband was depressed also said he was angry. There is a high correlation between substance abuse and depression, and, in males, the risk of heart disease is doubled.

Again, professional help is imperative.

ANTIDEPRESSANTS AND LOW LIBIDO

As mentioned in chapter 2, in 2005, 118 million prescriptions were written in the United States to counteract depression. Antidepressants can, literally, save lives. Unfortunately, many have the possibility of adverse side effects, all of which your doctor should discuss with you. One of these is ironic: antidepressants may significantly lower an already low libido. In addition, they may cause erectile dysfunction, inhibited ejaculation, and/or anorgasmia (inability to achieve orgasm).

New medications to counteract depression are being developed on a regular basis, and scores are already on the market. Some (for most patients) have minimal sexual side effects, or none. A psychopharmacologist or psychiatrist determines the correct drug or combination of drugs by taking a medical history, through empirical trial and error, and/or with urine analysis. (A psychologist can diagnose, but cannot prescribe medication.) This is a highly specialized and individualized undertaking. There is no such thing as "one size fits all" when it comes to the vast number of different drugs available to counteract depression; the expertise of a specialist is important. In addition, the correct drug or drug combination may alleviate symptoms but not remove the reasons for the depression. This is why counseling is usually recommended in addition to the medication(s).

Drugs known as SSRIs (selective serotonin reuptake inhibitors) prevent the removal of the neurotransmitter serotonin from the system, and thus, in theory, elevate mood. Some common brand names are Prozac, Zoloft, Paxil, and Lexapro. It may be necessary for a patient to take these; they may be the ones that work. However, they also are the drugs most likely to result in libido lowering and other negative sexual side effects. If the patient experiences those side effects (about 40% do), other medications may be substituted or the dosage may be reduced.

A newer group of drugs add norepinephrine and usually result in less of a negative effect on libido. These are referred to as SSNRIs (selective serotonin norepinephrine reuptake inhibitors). Some name brands are Cymbalta and Effexor. The side effects most likely to occur with these drugs are nausea, dizziness, and dry mouth, although erectile dysfunction and inhibited orgasm have been reported.

NDRIs (norepinephrine dopamine reuptake inhibitors) balance and boost those two neurotransmitters in the brain. The brand names are Wellbutrin and Wellbutrin XL. There seem to be limited adverse sexual side effects for NDRIs, although in a 2001 study, 20 percent of men taking the drug experienced some dysfunction. (Interestingly, the drug is currently being researched as a libido enhancer for women.)

Numerous other drugs are available, all with different molecular structures and effects on the brain—far too many to discuss here. We have touched briefly on the most widely prescribed. We want the reader to be aware that there are options, that it is necessary for an expert to help men choose the correct option, and that it is important to ask questions about possible side effects. Your family doctor may help you navigate your choices of mental health specialists, and give referrals, but is unlikely to be able to adequately sift through all of the possible drugs to make the best choice for you or your spouse.

It is important to remember that clinical depression is a serious and potentially fatal disease and should be treated as such. A depressed person's lack of libido is in no way a reflection of his feelings for his partner; it is a result of the illness and/or, quite possibly, the medication to cure it.

It is worth noting that of the men who strongly agreed they were depressed, 46 percent said they were taking medication that lowered their libido.

Not surprisingly, 82 percent of the men who took what they perceived as libido-lowering medication for *any* physical condition reported erectile dysfunction, rapid ejaculation, or difficulty achieving orgasm.

CAN ANTIDEPRESSANTS CAUSE RELATIONSHIP BLUES?

SSRIs may do more harm to a relationship than just ending desire. Antidepressants may diminish feelings of romantic love and attachment, possibly even making a person feel that he is no longer in love. And if patients are often not told about the potential loss of libido, they are just about never told about the possible inability to experience romantic love. Anthropologist Helen Fisher, who has done extensive research on the chemistry of love, told us that when SSRIs elevate the level of serotonin in the synapses of the brain, they suppress the dopamine circuits. These are the circuits that are activated when you fall madly in love. They're what make you want to be with your beloved every moment, and despair if you're not. They are also what cause you to sexually crave your new love with an intensity that will rarely, if ever,

Antidepressants may diminish feelings of romantic love and attachment.

be recaptured after those first few months or years. Dr. Fisher believes that if you elevate serotonin, you tamper with the brain system that allows you to fall in love and stay in love. She states: "We know that the reason people take SSRIs is to blunt the emotions and to curb obsessive thinking and [these] are both central characters of romantic love. So, as you take the SSRIs you're blunting the emotions, you're suppressing the dopamine circuits, and you're trying to kill obsessive thinking. All three of those are primary to romantic love."

Thus, depression may lower libido, and so may some antidepressants. In addition, these same libido-lowering SSRIs may prevent a person from experiencing romantic love. That person may actually "fall out of love" while taking the medication, and have it come flooding back when weaned off the drug. These drugs may be necessary and have a positive result. At the same time, there may be some surprising, and not so positive, unintended consequences.

As far back as the 1955 musical *Silk Stockings,* Cole Porter had his beautiful Russian protagonist Ninotchka sing about desire with the cool skepticism of a communist agent, which she was. When the handsome American lead says he is madly in love with her, she cynically proclaims "It's a chemical reaction, that's all." Needless to say, she falls passionately in love by the time the curtain falls.

It may be odd to think of love and sex in terms of neurotransmitters, hormones, and chemical reactions. But recently, there has been much evidence of "chemistry" behind romance—lust hormonally driven by androgens and estrogens, the euphoria of new love by high levels of dopamine and norepinephrine and low levels of serotonin, and the serenity of long-term commitment by hormones oxytocin and vasopressin. It is therefore possible that unless a couple works hard at keeping those dopamine and norepinephrine levels high and all the other chemicals in balance, desire will fade.

Many other drugs have potentially negative sexual side effects, including but not limited to medications for blood pressure, heart disease, diuretics, and even certain antihistamines. Twenty-six percent of the female respondents agreed that their partners were taking medication that lowered their libido; 21 percent of the men said this was so. If you or your partner suspect a medication is causing sexual or any other type of problems, talk to your doctor. It may be possible to decrease dosage or switch to a different product.

eight

ERECTILE DYSFUNCTION: THE SILENT PASSION KILLER

I just don't seem to do it for him. In addition, when we do have sex, he isn't hard; this embarrasses him, so he doesn't even try anymore. **(Female, 36)**

I believe that his natural shyness and performance anxiety was exacerbated by repeated incidences of sexual dysfunction and eventually he just gave up on himself and stopped trying. **(Female, 50s)**

Men are supposed to be ready to go at the drop of a bra. Therefore, a lot of guys believe that the easy erections they had when they were 16 should keep on rising effortlessly at 60. You've probably all heard the one about a woman needing to build desire slowly, simmering like a Crock-Pot, while a man gets aroused in an instant, similar to nuking leftovers in a microwave. Although we never much liked the analogy, the Crock-Pot/microwave comparison has some truth to it. Women, as a rule, *do* take longer to reach a level of peaked desire and achieve orgasm. Men *are* often ready much sooner.

Only about 20 percent of men with ED seek professional help.

However, some women are ready to go at the speed of light, some men need a lot of stimulation, and sex, like life, is often surprising. But it should be no surprise if a man needs more stimulation as he ages, because many do. Multiple studies have indicated a decline in male sexual functioning after age 40. In spite of this, when Lenore Tiefer interviewed hundreds of men at Montifiore Medical Center in the Bronx, she found that most of them expected to get an erection just by looking at nude pictures in *Playboy,* and this included men in their 50s. The expectation that erections will come as easily at 60 as 16 is irrational. Nearly four out of ten baby boomers report that they or their partners have experienced erectile dysfunction, something likely to be underreported. Statistics vary, solutions vary, but the websites of the big three erectile dysfunction drugs—Viagra, Cialis, and Levitra—all agree on one thing: ED affects over 30 million men in the United States. Validating studies, including the 1992 National Health and Social Life Survey, report the same figure. This is a serious problem, and not to be overlooked or dismissed, although many men choose to do so. Frequently it can be easily and effectively cured, if the man is willing to admit there's a problem. Bob Dole and famous athletes endorse ED drugs, and the back walls of baseball stadiums scream VIAGRA. Nevertheless, only about 20 percent of men with ED seek professional help.

HOW ERECTION OCCURS

When physical or mental stimulation results in the brain sending a message of arousal via the nervous system to the penis, here's what (ideally) happens: The artery to the penis dilates to twice its diameter, blood flow is increased, and the veins that carry blood away from the penis are blocked. The two spongy, cylinder-shaped structures in the shaft of the penis called corpora cavernosa relax, allowing the increased flow of blood to cause expansion. A membrane surrounds the corpora cavernosa, which helps to trap the blood and sustain erection. Thus, an erection takes place when there is increased inflow and decreased outflow of blood to the penis. (This can also happen on an involuntary basis due to friction, or upon awakening, or during sleep.)

There are seemingly endless erectile variations other than the ideal. A man may be unable to achieve erection on a temporary or more permanent basis, or get a partial one, or get one and lose it several times while making love, or get one but not maintain it for intercourse, or initially maintain it for intercourse but not sustain it. The experience may be elusive, with numerous permutations, or always pretty much the same. But unless there is increased inflow and decreased outflow of blood to the penis, no erection takes place.

WHAT PREVENTS AN ERECTION?

Blood has to flow easily into the penis, and remain trapped there for a period of time, to enable it to become erect. Therefore, vascular diseases, such as arteriosclerosis (hardening of the arteries) or high cholesterol (excess cholesterol adheres to artery walls, making it difficult for blood to pass through) can impede an erection. Heart disease and stroke may also have a negative effect. Other physical causes include diabetes, and the aftermath of colon, rectal, or prostate surgery. In addition, many medications have ED as a possible side effect, including some for depression, anxiety, diabetes, and hypertension. Any of the above, in relation to optimal sexual health, should be discussed with a physician as soon as possible.

Lifestyle factors can also diminish a man's ability to get or maintain an erection. As almost everyone has experienced at least once, too much alcohol rarely leads to a great night of passion. A heavy drinker may experience erectile dysfunction on a more permanent basis. Drug abuse also can discourage an erection (and a partner). So can obesity. Healthier men have an easier time getting and maintaining erections, and eating less and exercising more can result not only in weight loss, but in better sex. Clearly, poor lifestyle choices are often indicators of other psychosocial factors, and the cause of physiological ones. And anything as serious as alcoholism, drug abuse, or obesity should be dealt with immediately, ED or not. But potency can be an additional benefit of improved habits.

THAT MAGIC WAND: HOW CAN A MAN COMPETE?

When Hitachi developed a microphone-shaped vibrating "massage therapy" product that became the bestselling vibrator of all time, they called it a Magic Wand. It was a supernatural pleasure tool— only a blackout could impede performance. Men are conditioned to believe that they should perform, for better or for worse, in sickness and in health, just like that appliance. They should turn on as soon as the switch is pushed, and keep on going, even if 30 million of them don't.

Men are conditioned to believe that they should perform, for better or for worse, in sickness and in health.

Why is there so much denial of a problem that affects so many? Urologist Abraham Morgentaler states that shame is the primary reason men do not seek help: "They are ashamed they cannot perform sexually the way they once did or think they should." To compound the problem, many think the cause is psychological, even though it more often isn't. "Persistent failure then becomes a sign (in their own minds) of failed willpower in addition to a failed erection—another sign of diminished masculinity." Journalist David M. Friedman argues that there aren't too many ways left for a man to prove that he is protective and strong, as technology has robbed him of most easy displays of male prowess. "A man is no longer measured by his physical strength, his ability to build shelter for his family, fight in hand-to-hand combat, or draw water from a well. Machines do that for him. Muscles are more symbolic than useful. So the erect penis has become the most powerfully symbolic muscle of them all." Sociologists suggest that the past thirty years challenged men's traditional areas of supremacy tremendously—they were no longer necessarily the most powerful sex at home, work, or in politics. Erectile dysfunction may be the last, limp straw—the ultimate threat to an already shaky masculinity.

Of course, a loss of the ability to get or maintain an erection can be sliced and diced into a million sociological, physiological, and psychological pieces—but when it happens to a man it is devastating. There used to be little reason *not* to suffer in silence; what's the point of discussing this with your physician if you don't think there's any cure? Then, in March of 1998, just weeks after Monicagate broke and the president of the United States's penis and semen began to be discussed regularly on the nightly news, Viagra was approved by the FDA and became a household word. The "little blue pill" wasn't just a boon to the millions of men who needed some help, but to late-night talk-show hosts, too. (We can't blame them for making jokes, it's what they get paid for, but can you imagine anyone laughing about a new pill that cured diabetes or heart disease?)

If you suffer from ED, it's hardly a joke, and finally there was a solution other than embarrassingly awkward penile pumps, surgery, questionable herbs, unappealing suppositories, and even less appealing injections. And miraculously, the little blue pill worked for most men. That is, if they were among the 20 percent courageous and secure enough to give it a try.

ANOTHER UNFORTUNATE MALE EQUATION:
NO ERECTION = NO SENSE OF SELF

He doesn't get much of an erection and feels like he is a failure as a husband. (Female, 66, married to her 66-year-old husband for five years)

J. Francois Eid is a New York City urologist specializing in erectile dysfunction. He believes that if a man loses his potency, he loses a part of his identity. Essayist Phillip Lopate agrees—he quips that just saying the word out loud makes him nervous. Sociologist Warren Farrell once mentioned that it is a rare disease that *becomes* the identifying characteristic of the inflicted, as in "I *am* impotent," in contrast to, for example, "I *have* cancer." This seems to be the case in sexual issues, regardless of gender. A woman is likely to say that she is nonorgasmic, and it wasn't too long ago that nonorgasmic women were called "frigid." Similarly, the extreme negativity of *not* being potent resulted in a new, politically correct way of stating the case; around 1992, it became known as erectile dysfunction, or ED for short, allowing Tom Wolfe to wittily call impotence "the disease that dares not speak its name."

An ego-threatening disease by any other name is still a marital landmine.

Many men shut down completely, afraid that kissing and other displays of affection might be misconstrued and lead to embarrassment. It is easier to pretend fatigue, or (not necessarily duplicitously) claim anxiety and stress and far less threatening to masturbate and get a release of tension—no erection necessary. Some men shut down so completely that erectile dysfunction inhibits their ability to feel any desire at all. A 1990 study found that 20 percent of men who experienced ED also had a difficult time having an orgasm.

To compound the problem, it is usually extremely difficult if not impossible for a woman to understand how devastating this is. Even the most sophisticated woman, in terms of male sexual function, may irrationally blame herself, believing she is no longer attractive, desirable, or loved. When conventional solutions like new lingerie and candlelit bubble baths fail miserably, she may become angry, depressed, or both. It is understandable for a woman to be frustrated, confused, or even enraged when she feels less than desirable; it is also not surprising that some suspect their partners of infidelity. However, so many men suffer from this problem that it is important to realize that although no one wants to talk about it, maybe least of all your spouse, you are not alone. You are part of a silent crowd.

VIAGRA, CIALIS, AND LEVITRA ARE NOT, WE REPEAT *NOT*, APHRODISIACS

We must mention here that those blue, yellow, and orange pills, respectively, do not cause a man to become excited. They only work if he is aroused, and the arousal part will only happen if he is "turned on" by his partner or some other stimulation. We cannot state this too strongly. It is easy for us to understand why some women feel disappointed that their partners need a pill to get an erection, but it is not a rational disappointment. In fact, these pills can be an easy solution to a problem that was once extremely difficult to solve.

Pills won't give men an erection unless they are stimulated. They have zero effect on low libido.

So, one more time, pills won't give men an erection unless they are stimulated. They have zero effect on low libido. A guy who is willing to ask for help from his doctor is taking a big, difficult step and is really trying to solve the problem. If the problem is physical, and it usually is, PDE5 drugs (short for phosphodiesterase type 5) work 65 percent of the time.

Pfizer's Viagra (sildenafil), Lilly's Cialis (tadalafil) and Bayer's Levitra (vardenafil) all work in more or less the same way, by allowing blood vessels to relax enough to increase the flow of blood to the penis and stay there. Although all are similar compounds, they have small molecular differences, which mean that if one proves unsuccessful, another might work just fine.

Viagra takes about one hour to work and lasts about four. It should be taken on an empty stomach; doctors suggest three hours after eating.

Cialis takes about thirty minutes to work and lasts about thirty-six hours, which is why the pill is called "Le Weekend" in France. It can be taken with or without food. (Full disclosure: Bob has been a spokesperson for Cialis.)

Levitra takes about forty-five to sixty minutes to become effective, lasts about four hours, and can be taken with or without food.

They all may interact with other medications, so the physician will need a complete list of any being used. He will probably recommend alternatives to the PDE5s if the patient suffered a heart attack or stroke in the past six months, has very high or low blood pressure, liver or kidney disease, or certain other, less common physical conditions.

The physician will help decide the most appropriate pill. For example, diabetics, with a slower rate of gastric emptying, might be advised to use Cialis or Levitra because they can be taken with food.

He might also recommend you consult a urologist.

Confidence Resurrection

We mentioned that these pills aren't love potion number nine. However, if a man stops being sexual with his partner because of ED and ED only, and takes a pill that alleviates the problem, he may be able to make love again eagerly and fearlessly. He still has to get aroused, but a renewed belief in himself and his sexual abilities may enable passion to come back along with his erection.

What If the Pills Don't Work?

For men with psychological impotence and without additional physiological factors, the efficacy rate is 80 percent; as previously stated, this decreases to about 65 percent for men with physical causatives and 50 percent for men with severe medical conditions such as a combination of diabetes and hypertension. The drugs most commonly fail in men over 60 with severe insulin-dependent diabetes or impaired arterial blood flow. There are other reasons why these drugs don't have an even higher success rate. Some men simply use them incorrectly, for example, by taking Viagra on a full stomach.

> He is only 40 and the fact that neither Viagra nor Cialis worked suggests to me that something else is going on and he's not telling me. This is just my guess. I have snooped all over the house and have found nothing illicit, but I just can't believe the ED drugs didn't work for any reason. The lack of intimacy is killing my spirit. I don't even feel like a woman anymore. (Female, 30s)

It concerns us that a woman might think she is the reason the pills aren't working. After all, he can't get an erection—that's ego deflating enough. Then, he takes a pill that's supposed to give him one, and *that* doesn't work. It can seem like the end of the road, incontrovertible proof that her husband no longer finds her attractive, when the truth is that the medicine is unfortunately ineffective in his case. We mentioned earlier that it is extremely difficult for a woman to realize the devastation a man likely feels if he experiences erectile dysfunction, especially on a regular basis. It may be equally impossible for a man to understand how insecure his partner feels if he doesn't get an erection even after taking a pill.

It is extremely important to remember the statistics here. These drugs are not infallible, and the reason they don't work is probably because they are the wrong medication for the situation; they simply aren't improving blood flow to the penis. While it is true that a man may no longer find his partner attractive, and a man may fall out of love, that probably isn't a man who will take a pill in an attempt to reactivate his sex life. Conversely, a man may adore his wife and find her irresistible, but not be able to achieve an erection, even with that pill.

If the drugs prove ineffective, there are other paths to explore, including implant surgery, penile suppositories, revascularization (reestablishment of blood supply) and injection therapy. And although the ED drugs are most often prescribed by a family physician, if they fail and incorrect usage is not the reason, the urologist should most certainly be consulted.

We strongly suggest a couple visit doctors together to learn about the PDE5s' correct usage and efficacy rate, and to explore alternative options if they don't work. We don't suggest this is easy, but, realistically, it's not that difficult, either. Men just have to get over their fear of impotency making them less of a man—if that were true, there wouldn't be that many "real men" around over the age of 40—and women have to get past thinking that the pills are getting him aroused and she's not. If there is ever a time in a marriage to each put the other's feelings first, and to try and imagine what your partner is going through, this is it.

SEXUAL INTIMACY

Many of the metaphors for penis (rod, battering ram, and wand, for example) reinforce the fantasy that a penis is always hard, stiff, and ready. Sociologist Susan Bordo recommends that we "rethink that term 'hard' as it relates to the penis. When we imagine the erect penis as 'hard' we endow it with armor. . . . The penis, far from being an impenetrable knight in armor, in fact wears its heart on its sleeve. That's what's so magical about it."

Wouldn't it be fantastic to do this, to rethink "rock hard" as being mandatory for pleasurable sex? A less than firm erection might even be a positive thing, as Abraham Morgentaler elegantly suggests: "Curiously, some women have found that the man's inability to achieve a firm erection provides an opportunity for a different type of connecting: one in which the man is more vulnerable and in some ways more accessible to them emotionally. Being accepting of the man, whether or not he is 'performing well,' can unleash in him a flood of warm, positive feelings, which is likely to cause warmth and firmness in the penis as well." These words can be applied to all aspects of a truly intimate relationship; simple "acceptance" of a less than perfect situation can sometimes create something wonderful.

*A man's lack of an erection may feed
his partner's insecurities.*

The penis is a delicate, vulnerable, and, yes, magical organ. Its very lack of predictability is what makes it so exciting; it is attached to a living being with emotions, fears, self-doubts, and the ability to love and be loved. And although it may perform on command when a guy is 18, it isn't necessarily as reliable in later years. This often happens to a man just as his wife is going through menopause with all of the emotional and physiological baggage that accompanies the euphemistically labeled "change of life." She may not be feeling too sexy in our youth-oriented culture. (For example, when Larry King interviewed a widowed Candice Bergen about dating, she said that her age made her "invisible"— this from a tall, blond, beautiful, and, at the time, fiftysomething star.)

A man's lack of an erection may feed his partner's insecurities.

especially in midlife when ED is most likely causing cracks in otherwise solid marriages, and the problems of impotence may compound exponentially.

And so, acceptance can be the most intimate and rewarding gift a couple can give each other at this time. Then, they can work together toward a solution.

ED IS RARELY ONE-DIMENSIONAL

Sometimes a couple starts out trying to solve the problem with intelligence and tact, but then ego and foolish choices undermine success. A woman whose husband stopped being sexual with her when they were in their 30s (they have been together since college and married for ten years) states:

> Before things went sour we openly communicated about not wanting our relationship to become stagnant like other couples we knew. *[Up to that point, sex was]* pretty good. He was overly sexual until the decline and he is attractive, in shape, and very powerful in the workplace. Of course, in the early years everything is better and more frequent.

When sex became a rarity and infidelity was suspected, she went through his briefcase and discovered evidence that he had been using an escort service when out of town on business. She also found pornographic material and condoms. Angry and hurt by the betrayal but still in love with her husband, they entered therapy, and then saw a physician. (Many men are reluctant to see a therapist, especially for impotence; this man seemed eager, at first, to improve the situation.)

> I still had extreme feelings and couldn't leave the marriage. Communication got better, but sex hasn't in the short or long

term. My husband can't get it up, for me, anyway. We went to a doctor and he got all the pills—Viagra, Cialis, and Levitra. I cannot tell you the feeling I have when my husband has to take a pill so he can touch me. It hurts to the core. I've built a wall now and have become quite numb to the whole thing.

This woman is understandably upset. She has been let down twice, first by her husband, and then by a pill. She won't allow herself to understand what seems obvious: her husband doesn't need a pill to touch her; he needs a pill to prevent embarrassment. He would not be aroused unless he was stimulated, and it is extremely possible that her "numbness" stops him from being fully aroused even then. Indeed, she goes on to say that the pills: "only work once in a while." She also mentions that even if he gets an erection strong enough for penetration, he will lose the erection but continue the intercourse. "That does zero for me," she says.

When asked if her husband is ever interested in being sexual in ways that didn't require an erection, she answered: "Nope. He has kissed me probably a handful of times in the past year, but always a substance evoking it, not while sober, ever." And when questioned as to why her husband is no longer sexual with her, she is mystified. "Boredom, career moves, stress. Honestly, I'm just making things up. I really don't know."

Here is a successful man terrified of failure in this part of his life. Clearly, he still has desire when performance anxiety is omitted, thus his choice of escort service and masturbation. It is possible that a physical condition caused his ED, embarrassing him so much he shut down with his partner, and it compounded when he was given pills that only occasionally work. His wife, who takes tremendous pride in her appearance ("I'm attractive, 5'8", 130–135 lbs., with six-pack abs, 36C breasts, and long hair"), is devastated, believing she is no longer desired by her husband, not even with the aid of medication. So a man who thrives on success is giving up sex with his attractive partner to eliminate the possibility of failure, and a woman who needs reassurance about her looks is unwilling to accept a penis that is anything less than a battering ram as proof that she is still sexy and loved.

Anger, tension, job insecurity, financial or family problems—any of these can prevent a man from functioning in an optimal way.

There is no mention of the couple ever seeing a urologist to determine why a 36-year-old once "overly sexual" man in "good shape" would suddenly stop making love to his attractive wife. They were willing to see a therapist and a physician, and yet do not seem to be going any further to solve the problem, possibly because they are each too caught up in their personal angers, resentments, self-doubts, and fears. They are choosing resignation rather than acceptance. When asked about the future, the woman states: "I think about divorce a lot; however, we get along great, have great friends, and a great life. Is sex worth throwing it all away for? The time vested and deep care I have for him remains. I know he would do anything for me . . . well, almost, right?"

Anger, tension, job insecurity, financial or family problems—any of these can prevent a man from functioning in an optimal way. These problems can combine with medical conditions, prescription drugs, and lifestyle issues. ED is often a multidimensional problem. A 34-year-old woman told us:

He is a proud man, and the fact that he could not always function, or that I didn't have many orgasms with him, probably played into his decision [to stop having sex] quite a lot. But there were other problems, too. I think between my dissatisfaction with him working thirteen or more hours a day, six days a week, and my dissatisfaction with our neighborhood, and his impotence—he just quit.

She poignantly adds:

A man seems to need to protect his ego in this area, but in doing so he risks making his wife feel angry and unloved. It is such a shame a man will let his marriage fall into ruin just to protect his own feelings.

MEN SPEAK UP ABOUT ED

With all the negativity, fear, and embarrassment that surround impotence, 30 percent of our male respondents still checked this box as a reason why they no longer have sex with their wives. Although we still think the figure may be even higher, we believe that it's positive almost one-third of the men would admit to ED, even anonymously. Perhaps there is a shift toward acceptance, as boomers turn 60. (Thirty-nine percent of the women said that their husbands suffered from erectile dysfunction.) Not surprisingly, very few of the men who reported having ED wanted to talk about it. Here are some who did.

As I got older, my own body did not respond as quickly as it had when I was in my 20s and 30s (I am now 61). She would pull me on top of her and say something like, "You can do this," but, discovering that I had little or no erection, she would say "See? You really don't want to!" and roll over. This sort of castrating behavior actually started around twenty years ago; I was still approaching her regularly, and she would sometimes say "You're getting too old for this." I have always been vigorous and in good health. (Male, 61)

It is possible that this man's impotence was initially the result of anger toward his wife, whom he appears to consider critical and disengaged. He also wrote that although she would occasionally "allow" him to perform oral sex, she refused to reciprocate.

ED has a profound effect on a man's confidence and can undermine a marriage that is otherwise functioning well.

And this 55-year-old divorced man says that both erectile dysfunction and premature ejaculation were major problems in his marriage, and they continue to be so now that he is alone:

> I am still having these problems and I am very hesitant to get into a relationship with ANY woman.

ED has a profound effect on a man's confidence and can undermine a marriage that is otherwise functioning well. If you are a man suffering from this issue, we can't urge you strongly enough to see your physician. And remember that impotence can be devastating to your partner, too. If you are a woman whose partner has the problem, encourage him to get help, and remind yourself that it is extremely unlikely that you are the cause.

RAPID EJACULATION

The Kinsey report on male sexuality, published in 1948, stated that 75 percent of men ejaculated within two minutes. However, some therapists suggest that PE (premature, or "rapid," ejaculation) only became a "problem" that needed treatment a few decades ago, when sexual pleasure for the other half of the team became truly worthy of consideration, and female enjoyment was tied into length of intercourse. The American Psychiatric Association defines rapid ejaculation as follows:

A. Persistent or recurrent ejaculation with minimal sexual stimulation before, on, or shortly after penetration and before the person wishes it. The clinician must take into account factors that affect duration of the excitement phase, such as age, novelty of the sexual partner or situation, and recent frequency of sexual activity.
B. The disturbance causes marked distress or interpersonal difficulty.
C. This is not due exclusively to the direct effect of a substance (e.g., withdrawal from opioids [narcotic pain managers]).

Rapid ejaculation has more recently been defined as when ejaculation happens in less than one minute and occurs before, or soon after, penetration into the vagina. The defining characteristic, however, is that the male has no control, and generally has deep feelings of inadequacy and shame after it occurs. Clearly, a man suffering from PE may have reason to prefer solitary to partnered sex. It is considered to perhaps be the most common male sexual complaint. Twenty-five percent of American men suffer from rapid (or premature) ejaculation.

---

25 percent of American men suffer from rapid (or premature) ejaculation.

Perhaps due to an older demographic, this did not seem to be an issue of primary importance to our respondents. Although, like ED, possibly underreported, only 16 percent of the men said premature ejaculation was a factor in their not having sex with their wives, although 20 percent of the woman believed it was. This 46-year-old woman expresses remorse over the way she treated her 45-year-old partner:

I'm sorry I let myself get so angry when he started to have a problem with premature ejaculation. I was so mad because he was pretending it wasn't a problem. I was so frustrated I used to yell at him after he had an orgasm.

Clearly, this woman's insensitivity to an issue her spouse considered extremely embarrassing compounded his anxiety, which, in turn, likely exacerbated the problem.

PE is one of the easiest sexual problems to solve, using behavioral therapy. A man can train his body to be aware of when he is getting close to the point of inevitability, and then either slow down or change what he's doing. Many men self-trained to be rapid ejaculators in those furtive and fast early days of adolescent masturbation and continue this behavior into adulthood. Then they try, unsuccessfully, to "retrain" by focusing on anything other than their partner and the sensations of lovemaking. They rationalize that if they think about baseball scores or interoffice memos, the problem will go away. The fallacy with this approach is that they are also "retraining" to be uninvolved, uncommitted partners, while doing nothing to decrease the performance anxiety that is the psychological foundation for rapid ejaculation. For example, a fear of intimacy or discomfort with his own sexuality can lead to PE; further separation from his sexuality might only aggravate the real issues. In addition, he may become so expert at this waiting game that erectile dysfunction replaces premature ejaculation as a different road to the same ultimate, sexless destination. He is doing nothing to reduce his stress and anxiety.

There has been some recent research, and preliminary success, in treating PE with low doses of antidepressants. The caveat, of course, is that it may treat the condition, but lower the libido. The erectile dysfunction drugs also have shown promise, and if premature ejaculation has been a problem, it is certainly worthwhile discussing both with your physician.

RETARDED EJACULATION

The inability to be orgasmic or just taking too long—these are usually seen as exclusively women's issues. Men having a problem ejaculating is rarely discussed. And yet 27 percent of our female respondents felt this was a reason their husbands stopped being sexual. Fifteen percent of the males agreed.

Numerous medications can cause a man to have this problem. These include some (but by no means all) drugs that treat cardiovascular issues. Many drugs for depression and anxiety that lower libido prevent or inhibit ejaculation as well. If necessary, discuss this with your physician. It may be possible to switch to a different medication, or reduce dosage. Substance abuse, especially cocaine and marijuana, can also result in inhibiting orgasm. One of our male respondents reported that although he no longer has his heroin addiction, he still has difficulty maintaining an erection or having an orgasm.

Male retarded ejaculation is rarely a psychological issue. However, it has been theorized that certain men are so anxious to please their partners that they are unable to relax enough to please themselves, similar to some nonorgasmic females. Others can orgasm only with prolonged friction generally not possible during intercourse. These men can ejaculate when alone, or sometimes with manual partnered stimulation.

BETTER SEX THROUGH CHEMISTRY?

The pharmaceutical companies are researching new and improved drugs for male sexual issues, for example, the next generation of PDE5 inhibitors. A low-dosage "once-a-day" version of Cialis (2.5 mg as compared with current 5 mg, 10 mg, and 20 mg dosages now available) was approved for the European market. U.S. application has been submitted. This will be marketed as a pill for men who want to be able to function sexually at any time. They can, theoretically, take a pill every morning with their baby aspirin and vitamin, and love will truly mean never having to say they're sorry. If it works, the guy will once again be his old, pre-ED self.

SSRIs (selective serotonin reuptake inhibitors) have been prescribed off-label by physicians for years in the treatment of rapid ejaculation. Dapoxetine, an SSRI specifically developed to be marketed for this purpose, was recently rejected approval by the FDA but was granted it in Europe. In one study, although Dapoxetine was perhaps not as efficacious as one might hope (the participants were able to have intercourse for an additional minute), those taking it did report more enjoyment and control over their performance. As we have previously mentioned, SSRIs, marketed as antidepressants, can result in lower libido, erectile dysfunction, and inhibited orgasm (hence the off-label usage for rapid ejaculation). A new generation of SSRIs is being researched to treat depression without deleterious sexual side effects.

Hormonal birth control for men appears to be in the not too distant future. A progestin-releasing implant will be effective for up to a year when combined with quarterly injections of androgen and is reversible. For the first time, men who fear impregnating their partners, perhaps to the point of not being able to optimally function, will be in complete control, without having to disrupt the sex act in any way.

Lifestyle drugs can be extremely effective and can, in fact, have a significantly positive effect on one's life and style. But, if men don't use them, all the new innovative research won't make any difference. What angered so many of our female respondents was their husband's refusal to get any help for his problem of erectile dysfunction, when it seemed so readily available. According to them, seven out of ten men suffering from impotence refused to see a physician.

nine

CAUGHT IN THE NET

When we bought our computer over six years ago, our sex life started to go downhill. He would spend all night watching porn. I would lie in bed alone and wonder if he even loved me anymore. **(Female, 20s)**

We had some surprises while doing our research, but it was no shock that a woman takes it personally when her partner secretly masturbates to a virtual lover. It is both mysterious and hurtful that a beloved would prefer a solitary experience with a one-dimensional online fantasy to an intimate and real one with his wife.

Masturbation seems to play a different role in the sex lives of men and women. When Shere Hite compiled her two classic statistical volumes of male and female sexuality in the late 1970s, she noted that "most women felt that the main importance of masturbation was to substitute for sex (or orgasm) with a partner," but "almost all men, whether married or single, with or without an otherwise active sex life, said they made masturbation a regular part of their lives."

He once told me that he likes to masturbate because he can focus on himself and he doesn't have to worry about pleasing another person. He knows what he likes and he gets it done quickly. (Female, 20s)

Psychiatrist and sex therapist Avodah K. Offit, in her beautifully written *Night Thoughts: Reflections of a Sex Therapist,* says this about masturbation: "Whether we share our sexuality becomes a matter of choice, not obligation. Most men take this freedom for granted, but many women need to be taught," and then adds that, from a woman's perspective, "For most of us, the ultimate message of masturbation is still a longing for someone else."

This seems to be an irreconcilable difference. In spite of all the childhood taboos or because of them—the subterfuge, fear of being caught, parental warnings and recriminations—most men seem to make time for masturbation whether they're in a relationship or not. It's simply a question of how much time and energy they have left for partnered sex.

If most men consider masturbation a birthright, it seems clear that a daily groaning board of sexual fantasies to help them along, virtually endless in variety, private, and cheap, would have appeal. The audience laughs loudly and knowingly in the musical *Avenue Q* when a female puppet sings the praises of the Internet for easy access to information and online shopping, but a cynical male puppet retorts: "Why do you think the Internet was born? Porn, porn, porn!"

There is plenty of porn to go around, with or without the Internet. America is the world's largest producer of "adult entertainment"—an estimated $10 billion industry. Dr. Joy Browne, psychologist and radio personality, says that although the Internet has changed accessibility, "Porn is as old as the cave painting. The only thing to change is the technology, not the phenomenon."

Nevertheless, easy access has possibly increased time spent with pornography for those guys once limited to line drawings and erotic stories. Fifty-eight percent of the men who responded to our survey said they watched porn online regularly. Of that group, 72 percent watched one to five hours per week, 19 percent six to ten hours per week, and 9 percent amazingly watched more than eleven hours a week, which would translate to a minimum of twenty-three days a year. They did not say, however, that pornography was necessarily the primary reason they stopped being sexual with their wives, and it might have been the result of marital problems rather than the cause.

A lot of "women of the night" have been replaced by "women of the Web."

Thirty-nine percent of the women reported that their husbands watched pornography online regularly. Of that group, 67 percent reported one to five hours weekly, 19 percent six to ten hours, and 13 percent said more than eleven hours a week.

Of course, the women could only approximate, and their anger and frustration may have inflated those estimates. Conversely, the men may not be aware of how much time they are really spending with their private harem of gorgeous smiling women who will never reject them or ask for anything that can't be delivered. What a place! To paraphrase Garrison Keillor—all the women are beautiful, all the men are hard, and all the sex is above average.

HOW CAN A WOMAN COMPETE WITH A DREAM?

Before pornography was readily available and "proper" women saved themselves for marriage (or at least a commitment), sex often appeared at the top of young men's shopping lists. Nineteenth-century men learned about how to please a woman by visiting prostitutes, and they were taught a wildly inaccurate view of female sexuality in the process. Swiss psychiatrist Auguste Henri-Forel warned about this when he said: "The company of prostitutes often renders men incapable of understanding feminine psychology, for prostitutes are hardly more than automata trained for the use of male sensuality. When men look among these for the sexual psychology of women they find only their own mirror."

Although a lot of "women of the night" have been replaced by "women of the Web," this remains a terrific depiction of what twenty-first-century DVDs and online pornography delivers, and if a man confuses it with real life, it can create serious problems. In *Mismatch: The Growing Gulf Between Women and Men*, political scientist Andrew Hacker, crunching the numbers in search of answers to the question of why "marriages are briefer than at any time since this nation began" suggests that, as example, the large market for pornography "conveys a lot about what men want—and apparently aren't getting—from their marriages."

I'd just like to reiterate that this is one of the worst problems that a relationship can go through. Now that I have left my pornographically obsessed ex-husband I have realized how emotionally abusive it is to withhold sex and still demand that your partner be monogamous. I think a lot of people assume that this type of situation only occurs when women have had a bunch of kids or are not as physically attractive as they once were. At the time I was 23 years old, in very good shape, and described as very attractive. My ex-husband, for whatever reason—I think laziness—was still more interested in looking at pictures online than interacting with a real live woman who he claimed he loved. (Female, 20s)

remark. "Always with the same hen?" he inquires. "Heck no," his guide replies, "a different one every time." To which the president says, with a wink, "Be sure to tell that to Mrs. Coolidge."

For some men pornography is supplemental sex, a way of getting variety into their lives without cheating.

For some men pornography is supplemental sex, a way of getting variety into their lives without cheating. Online, a man can rule the roost, at least in his imagination. Some wives may be fine with this, especially if husbands bring it back to the bedroom. As a woman in her 20s said wistfully: "If watching porn could get him aroused, I'd be all for it."

Dr. Reinisch recommends trying to understand why your partner is choosing to do this, and turning it around to make it something you do together. For example, even if a woman would never consider doing what her husband fantasizes about online, she might consider dressing up in something sexy and watching by his side, instead of shutting him out. She suggests: "You can't do things that are against your values, but you might be able to get to the point where you can have sex with him while he's watching sometimes. Not all the time; then that's not fair." In this way, her husband gets his imaginary world, along with his real woman. She cautions that putting a label on his actions may produce a negative effect. "By saying it's an addiction, in other words causing him to feel wrong, sick, and dirty, you push him away." She adds that it should be a signal to a woman that something is wrong in the relationship, because, she believes, any man who is feeling good about himself will prefer a live woman to an imaginary one, but if he thinks demands are being made of him he can't deal with or fulfill, he might turn to a computer screen.

Reinisch, of course, is speaking about women aware of their husbands' activities, and even perhaps willing to join them. Online erotica may become a temporary bridge back to a healthy sex life far away from cyberspace. It may also add some seasoning and zest occasionally or on a more regular basis; these are intimate negotiations only a couple can broker.

However, there are wives who know that their husbands are viewing porn and consider it not a misdemeanor or even a felony, but an abomination. Dr. Julian Slowinski is a senior clinical psychologist at Pennsylvania Hospital and has been on the faculty of the University of Pennsylvania School of Medicine for more than twenty-five years. He told us that he once had a woman say that looking at *Playboy* was adulterous. Sex therapist Max Fitzgerald, who administers couple's therapy along with his wife, Della Fitzgerald, said: "We've had a number of men believe that they were committing adultery because they fantasized about someone other than their wife. If you interpret the Bible literally, Christ said, 'you are as guilty for the thought as you are for the deed.'" The Fitzgeralds said they worked with several men who were so guilty about fantasizing during sex with their wives, they stopped being sexual in any way whatsoever—they "pulled the plug on eroticism." There are certainly those who, for cultural or religious reasons, think viewing pornographic material to be adulterous and therefore sinful. If a man feels compelled to watch online erotica, he may shut down completely rather than allow himself to do something he considers wicked, in his mind, heart, or bed. As Max Fitzgerald says about passionate sex: "Guilt will kill it in a heartbeat."

What is acceptable or not is personal and unique and should be respected. If one partner or both partners feel that viewing pornography or fantasizing in other ways is a sin, but one still feels compelled to do so or is married to someone who does, it would likely be beneficial to speak to a therapist or member of the clergy. The issue, however, may be based not on religion but on feelings of exclusion and loss of trust, especially if the partner discovers the online "cheating" accidentally. In that case, if it is at all feasible, it is probably far better to use those fantasies as playful, private erotica.

That is, of course, if they are within both individuals' area of comfort. To be simplistic, if a woman dislikes performing oral sex and her husband craves it, it is likely that he will fantasize about it a great deal, and perhaps decide to watch a woman perform fellatio online and masturbate rather than ask his wife and get rejected one more time. The fellatio-averse woman might find it acceptable, however, to join her husband in his online fantasy world as a compromise. When Bob wrote *His Secret Life: Male Sexual Fantasies,* he discovered that most men want adventures just slightly out of the ordinary (e.g., sex out of doors or light S&M) and that more often than not, if the fantasy involved two women, one of them was his wife. The book was published in 1997, with fantasies collected from 1994 to 1996, just prior to Internet sex becoming ubiquitous.

Dr. Bob Mendelsohn theorizes that sexual fantasies are determined early in life and unlikely to change. Gerald Weeks and Nancy Gambescia would disagree. They believe fantasies do change over time, influenced, in their clinical experience, by "what is portrayed in the media, especially pornography." It is possible that fantasies will be radically altered by the ever-expanding and bar-raising quality of online pornography. Research to determine the effects of the Internet on male sexuality is just beginning.

CAN WATCHING ONLINE PORNOGRAPHY BE ADDICTIVE?

He doesn't smoke, drink, or gamble, but he spends hours a day downloading pornography. He may be wasting a lot of time, but is he an addict?

Although Internet addiction disorder has not yet been recognized as a psychiatric diagnosis, therapists report working with numerous patients for whom sexual activity is considered to be uncontrollable. Some consider Internet addiction to be growing so rapidly they regard it as an epidemic. Sandra Leiblum and Raymond Rosen, in the introduction to their third edition of *Principles and Practice of Sex Therapy,* state that what they believe to be "most worrisome" about online pornography is "individuals prone to sexually compulsive behavior who find the lures of cyberspace appealing."

The *New York Times* reports that approximately 6 percent to 10 percent of the estimated 189 million Internet users in America are addicted to the Web, although not necessarily to online pornography. Hilarie Cash runs Internet/Computer Addiction Services in Microsoft's hometown of Redmond, Washington. She and other therapists believe compulsive masturbatory fantasy can intensify due to the pervasive quality of the Internet, and that healthy people can be lured into addiction. She adds that her patients often struggle with other issues, like depression and anxiety.

The late Dr. Al Cooper, a sex therapist in the San Jose Marital Services and Sexuality Center in San Jose, California, even assigned a number—watching eleven hours per week or more makes you an addict. Julian Slowinski believes that the word *addict* is overused and often incorrect, but he notes that he has had patients compelled on a daily basis to rush home, watch pornography, and then rush back to the office and work late in order to catch up, adding: "If a person's compulsive behavior is affecting his life, his job, and his marriage, that fits my definition." (Incidentally, because neither sex addiction nor Internet addiction are considered to be psychiatric diagnoses, "impulse control disorder" is frequently what therapists use when they write the bill. Otherwise the patient would pay out of pocket.) Ken Search told us that there are two broad categories of addicts: one goes from one partnered encounter to the next without any emotional involvement; the other has solitary sex almost exclusively, sometimes accompanied by compulsive masturbation.

Jay Parker is a chemical dependency counselor at the Internet/ Computer Addiction Services. He believes that pornography addicts suffer from a combination of emotional immaturity, lack of discipline, and a fear of intimacy, and that the Internet has changed things in the world of compulsive solitary sex and is growing rapidly because it has what he calls "the three A's: accessibility, affordability, and anonymity." He adds: "It's not your father's porn, where he looked at a centerfold."

A survey respondent who describes himself as a recovering sex addict told us:

> I was into kinky stuff, like bondage and S&M, and heavily into porn at the same time. I really did fit the profile of an addict. I took risks that could have cost me my job and my marriage. I never was with a prostitute and I've never had an affair. I never did any of this stuff with another person, even before marriage. I was terrified of STDs and very shy. I have occasional relapses where I'll download some porn, but those days are getting rare. (Male, 30s)

Some men painfully put their wives in an untenable position, even if they offer to watch alongside their partners. The following woman said that her husband stopped being sexual with her, viewed pornography for about ten hours a week, and visited strip clubs.

> The lack of libido is hard enough to deal with but the fact that he's more interested in online porn than me is a real slap in the face. I'm 32, attractive, size 4-6, have a good personality, and am quite adventurous in bed, so I find it all so difficult to understand. I think he puts women in categories—good and bad. He says he respects me too much to watch porn with me. (Female, 30s)

In a follow-up interview, she mentions that her husband was raped by a male neighbor when he was 8 years old. Being raped, especially as a child, is a trauma of such enormous consequence that it often results in the feeling of losing power over most, if not all, aspects of life. That would, of course, include sexuality. To compound the problem, he recently lost his job. This man feels he lost the ability to be in charge of his life when he was eight, and it's only getting worse. In his mind, online pornography may be the one thing he has control over.

The following woman (54) has been married to her husband (54) for thirty-one years. In 1989, she found plastic garbage bags filled with pornographic videos and thinks that his "addiction" has been going on at least since then. She says that he suffers from both erectile dysfunction and premature ejaculation.

> My husband has a sexual addiction to online pornography, and this had been a factor throughout our marriage—magazines, videos, Internet. The breaking point came in 2005 when he lost his job due to "inappropriate use of the Internet" using a company-owned laptop. I've tried to "fix" things over the years . . . seduction, etc., but pornography always wins. Unfortunately, the loss of his job has killed all desire to ever resume intimacy. We live like roommates, and divorce is now financially impossible.

The impact of watching pornography appears to be a matter of degree. If a man gets temporarily captivated by some online pornography sites, and his wife finds out by confession, accident, or creative investigation, this can turn into something positive—a chance to express fantasies and desires that will add some variety to a perhaps otherwise perfunctory sex life. However, there are more extreme situations, like those above, where a man shuts down completely, avoiding anything but solitary sex. A man's penis is often a gauge of his physical and mental health. And if it can only function sexually when he is alone with his computer, it is a sign of something critically wrong.

NO ERECTION REQUIRED

It is not unusual for an impotent man to reject partnered sex to avoid embarrassment. An erection isn't necessary for orgasm, however, as sex therapist Julian Slowinski emphasized. He believes that erotic material can provide at least some outlet for pleasure when a man is otherwise choosing celibacy over potential failure. For example, a woman told us her husband stopped all intimacy with her because "he was depressed and had health issues that interfered with his sexuality," then added he was a regular viewer of online and DVD pornography. This 54-year-old woman is also married to a man who has ED:

> He used to be an attentive lover. Suddenly he became "too tired," and our lovemaking fell off. Now all he wants is oral sex, if anything at all. I found out he is addicted to Internet porn, and watches it right next to me when he thinks I'm asleep. Just this week I discovered he is soliciting cybersex online. I am beside myself—I love him dearly and I am devastated.

Elsewhere, we explore the psychological and physiological reasons why men develop erectile dysfunction, stressing that ED does not necessarily mean low libido. But if it does unfortunately and irrationally lead to an avoidance of partnered sex, online pornography can offer an alternative—women who are seemingly insatiable, yet always satisfied. (And when it's over, who cares if they are, anyway?) Or, more simply put, it's better than failure or nothing at all.

NO INTIMACY REQUIRED, EITHER

Although some couples may occasionally use sexual material available on the Internet to add some variety and spice things up a bit, others go online to avoid being intimate with their partners. As a female survey respondent puts it:

> Porn is his way to deal with sex without risking emotional intimacy. I think that he believes, deep down in his heart, that he is bad, even evil, and he is afraid to show that to anyone. Being intimate with me would make him too vulnerable. (Female, 30s)

Some men go online to avoid being intimate with their partners.

The following 32-year-old woman, married to her 36-year-old husband for less than five years, has offered to try and replicate what he likes online, but he's turned her down, possibly because of his embarrassment and shame about his sexual interests:

> He swears that pornography isn't a substitute for sex with me, but I think it is. There have been times when we have not had sex for a month and then I find out that he has been downloading porn every day. I have asked him what he gets from porn that he would like to do with me; I'm pretty open-minded. He can't tell me. I don't have a problem with my partner viewing porn from time to time without me, but I take offense when things have been wrong in our sex life for over two years and he does this. My gut instinct tells me he has a fear of intimacy, and I think it's also his way of asserting himself against me, as if he were saying "look who is in control now."

Many of the women in our survey told us that the marriage was very hot at the beginning, but it cooled down rapidly. In some of these situations, the men might have been so afraid when things were going well they had to pull back in order to avoid being vulnerable. Often men who are afraid of intensely committed relationships suffered a childhood trauma, the most usual being early loss of a parent through death or divorce. The traumatic experience becomes something to be avoided; and so, paradoxically, if the man loves his wife deeply, he may try to prevent the pain of future loss by rejecting her sexually and having one or multiple affairs. Phone sex used to be ideal for such a man and now Internet chat is even better, especially if he believes that virtual infidelity isn't cheating. He may be having "relationships" with several women, but they are superficial and interchangeable; he would suffer no pain if they ended. And although fearful of the consequences if his wife finds out, he thinks there is a good chance she would forgive him and stay because he has never really been unfaithful. Of course, he has never been committed, either, although if his secret activities are discovered by his partner and she agrees to stay, they may discover, with the help of therapy, that this crisis enriches their marriage. After all, the worst has happened and his love is with him still; the ability to be intimate may follow.

THE GREAT INSULATOR

Pornography can be a thick emotional buffer zone, separating a man from rejection, masking his insecurities and perceived inadequacies. When viewed in secret, there is probably shame, but also a lot of adrenaline-fueled excitement that comes from furtively entering this forbidden world. If a man believes his masculinity is diminished, pornography can restore some order to his life. It can give him control when his world seems spiraling out of it. There is a risk of being caught, but not for a serious crime. Indeed, it can be perceived as no-fault cheating.

The problem is, if it is done frequently and surreptitiously, it may or may not be infidelity, but it is most definitely cheating—preventing the couple from attaining an emotionally complete relationship. And, to be realistic, if the guy is over 40, secretly masturbating to orgasm will most likely prevent partnered sex; the refractory period is too long, and his wife too familiar, to bring about the Coolidge effect.

ten

NO SEX PLEASE,
WE'RE EATING

My wife was never thin but was attractive when we met. When I asked her to be my wife, I was honest and told her that her extra weight bothered me. I asked her to promise to try to lose it after we married. She agreed. It wasn't long before I realized she had little intention of doing anything about her weight. Soon after that the fighting began and really hasn't stopped. We have been married for twenty-three years and have had no sex whatsoever for the past fifteen years. **(Male, 50s)**

I lost forty pounds for our wedding in September 2004. We probably had sex at least ten times in the week after the wedding. I gained back the forty pounds in the last year. We have had sex only once in the past seven months. I think if the situation does not improve, I may leave. I feel that our connection is lost. **(Female, 30s)**

If a cigar is sometimes just a cigar, is a soft penis sometimes, well, just uninspired? Thirty-eight percent of the male respondents to our survey agreed that their wife had "gained a significant amount of weight," and this was as at least one of the reasons they were no longer interested in being sexual with her. They might be accurate, at least about the extra pounds. The latest data from the United States National Center for Health Statistics state that over 60 million adults over the age of 20 are obese, and that although the percentage of adults who are overweight but not obese has remained at a steady 32–34 percent since 1960, obesity has increased from 13 percent to 34 percent during the same time period. We are obsessed with thinness in a fat society, hoping to lose weight even as we're supersizing. If we do manage to remain fit, we're jubilant and maybe even a little smug. When female respondents described themselves as attractive, the adjective "slim" was the most common descriptive and single-digit dress sizes were announced with pride. Some seemed to believe their very "thinness" should be sufficient to elicit an erotic response from their partner, and they were puzzled if it didn't.

For many men excess weight prevents passion.

Some men either prefer a woman who is a bit heavier or don't consider extra pounds a deterrent to a healthy sex life, but for many men excess weight prevents passion. When we asked Dr. Julian Slowinski about men's sexual reaction to obesity in their partners, he mentioned that in his private practice this is something very difficult to deal with or to even bring up. A man might love his wife and be embarrassed that he doesn't have sex with her because she is no longer physically attractive to him, not something he can easily communicate. Although Slowinski believes every couple to be unique, when asked if a man not having sex with his wife because she is overweight is a cover-up for other issues he said yes, it can be, but "very often that's all it is." We were both skeptical and surprised at the large number of men who claimed that weight was a reason they stopped having sex with their partners, but we must infer that this really is the case at least some of the time. Indeed, Joseph LoPiccolo and Jerry Friedman, two leading sex therapists and researchers, state that "lack of attraction to partner, usually weight gain" can be a primary causative of male hypoactive sexual desire disorder.

It is important to distinguish obesity from being a few pounds overweight, which may in fact be a healthy weight in any culture not preoccupied with unrealistic images and goals. And it may seem insensitive to say that a woman's weight gain is the reason her partner has stopped being sexual with her (and ludicrous to say it if her husband has put on weight, too). But it also may be true.

HOW MUCH *SHOULD* YOU WEIGH?

Since 1998 the body mass index, or BMI, has been used to determine optimal weight. Dividing your weight in pounds by your height in inches squared, and multiplying the result by 704.5, will establish your BMI. Less than 18.9 is "underweight"; 19 to 24.9, "normal"; 25 to 29.9, "overweight"; and 30 and above, "obese." This is a fairly rigorous standard, not to mention complicated and almost impossible to remember. However, if you take out your calculator to determine your BMI and find that the number is over 30, you should consider losing weight for a wide variety of reasons. Hypertension, type II diabetes, heart disease, breast cancer, stroke, and erectile dysfunction are just some of the serious health issues exacerbated by obesity.

If impotence is a man's Achilles' heel, a woman's is weight gain.

But it probably isn't necessary to take out your calculator, or even to get on a scale. If you are overweight to the point of obesity, you know it. And, although it isn't a pleasant thought, it might mean that you are less desirable to your spouse than you once were, assuming you were thinner when you met. We are well aware how sensitive an issue this is, especially to women. If impotence is a man's Achilles' heel, a woman's is weight gain. It is extremely painful to think you are no longer desired by the man you love just because you don't fit his ideal body image.

> This has been the hardest three and a half years for me. I love my husband very much, and it would be hard for me to leave him. I want things back the way they used to be. I feel he does not find me attractive anymore because I have gained weight. (Female, 20s)

When we asked the woman in the preceding quote how much weight she had gained, she replied, "About 50 pounds, total. I have since lost 30 of that and I'm working on the rest."

We are aware that men put on weight, too, and are less appealing sexually because of it. However, we are unfortunately in a culture that puts more of a premium on female physical beauty than male.

In addition, and we have noted this elsewhere, but it is worth repeating, there has been recent evidence of a link between obesity and impotence.

WHY DO SOME WOMEN BECOME OBESE?

No one becomes seriously overweight or obese in a year, and the reasons for women gaining inappropriate amounts of excess weight are as varied as why men stop having sex. There are speculations about genetic predetermination, making obesity not inevitable but more likely, and hormonal imbalances. A recent Tufts University School of Medicine study following 820 men and women from childhood to young adulthood has linked a history of depression and anxiety to obesity in women, finding that females who developed depression at an early age weighed more as adults. In addition, they determined a possibility that some depressed women self-medicate with food, perhaps because carbohydrates elevate levels of serotonin, which are lowered by depression. (Young men identified as depressed did not gain weight.) One can certainly speculate that a woman whose husband stops showing affection and desire might become depressed and overeat, and the resulting weight gain can seem a reason, albeit the wrong one, for his lack of passion. Her elevated serotonin levels might possibly lower *her* libido, making her less receptive to his sexual advances, and so they are, in fact, each contributing to the lack of intimacy, while "blaming" the other. As one respondent said:

> He recently told me, after years of denying it, that he doesn't find me physically attractive anymore. The sex stopped even before I gained weight and after I went into my depression, I gained a lot of weight. I'm sure that has something to do with it, but not everything. I've recently lost twenty-five pounds and haven't noticed a change in his attitude toward sex. (Female, 20s)

The American Psychiatric Association does not link any psychiatric disorder to obesity, and it is therefore not listed in the *Diagnostic and Statistical Manual of Mental Disorders*. It has been theorized that female obesity is grounded in a rejection of all things feminine and, conversely, a rejection of men; a denial of being a sexual being or the opposite, an excuse to stop being one; a defense against pregnancy or a psychologically symbolic pregnancy; a result of personal trauma; or a self-punishing lack of motivational skills. However, no evidence-based proof exists that any of these contradictory psychological speculations are valid. Hilde Bruch, a psychiatrist and pioneer in the diagnosis and treatment of eating disorders, mentions that obese women often believe that to be "big" means to be more like a father than a mother—that is, stronger and more important, a desire to be neither man nor woman, but both. Greeks called this "the third sex."

This 46-year-old man speculates that his wife gained weight to guarantee rejection—a self-fulfilling prophecy:

> My gut feel is that she's living out a pattern in which she gets people to reject her. The weight gain seems to be a way for her to "create" the reality that I no longer find her attractive. Very destructive. That, and comments like "If I don't have sex for the rest of my life it will be too soon" followed by (almost in the next breath) "I really DO miss sex. Not sex with YOU, just sex." Very confusing.

The woman described in the preceding paragraph is revealing ambivalence about herself, her sexuality, and her weight. Her consistency is contradiction, and she uses cruel words to refuse her husband before he rejects her, which she is certain he will. Her husband is probably correct in stating her weight gain is for concealed and destructive reasons. In reality, they are both "living out a pattern," in that he doesn't seem to be suggesting she get help with her issues, preferring instead to live with the situation and feel oppressed.

Maybe It's the Food

Weight gain is simply the result of consuming too many calories and not exercising enough for too many years. Life is stressful, delicious food is comforting, and eating out, especially in fast-food restaurants, can easily push daily caloric intake over the top. It's amazing how easy it is to gain weight. There are 3,500 calories in a pound of fat. So, if you believe your weight to be perfect, but without realizing it eat just 20 calories a day more than you need (about the amount of calories in a teaspoon of sugar), you will have consumed an extra 7,280 calories in a year—a weight gain of two pounds. In five years, you will be ten pounds heavier. Of course, this is theoretical. No one, not the most avid calorie counter, can possibly take in the same amount of calories, plus 20, on a daily basis. But you can see how you can eat well, be really careful, and still gain a *little* weight, which is not particularly significant to anyone but yourself, and only then if you are consumed by fantastical images of beauty even as you have birthdays and babies. However, if you gain *ten* pounds in one year, and don't change negative eating/exercise habits, in a decade you might be morbidly obese and wonder why.

Maybe It's to Numb the Pain

I buried my sexual feelings with drinking and eating. The only sexual thoughts I had were in my dreams. (**Female, 60s**)

In the mid-1980s, marital therapist and former psychological director of Weight Watchers International Richard B. Stuart and his wife, Barbara Jacobson, conducted a national survey on women, weight, sex, and marriage. They had nine thousand responses. Women self-identifying as fairly to very happily married had an average weight gain of 18.4 pounds in the first thirteen years of marriage; those who claimed to be fairly to extremely unhappy gained an average of 42.6 pounds. (The unhappy women were, on average, five pounds heavier on their wedding day, which was believed to be statistically insignificant.) They did not offer a control study of weight gained by single people over the same time period. However, marriage may be hazardous to your waist, perhaps due to security and contentment, a perception that once married one can let go a bit because the game has been won, or because staying home and caring for young children can be tedious—with the one available and constant perk, a close proximity to the refrigerator. But why, Stuart and Jacobson asked, do unhappily married women gain more than two and a half times as much?

They theorized that the main reasons are one or more of the following:

To avoid sex with their partner.
To prevent flirtations that might lead to infidelity.
To justify the abuse in a physically or psychologically abusive relationship.
To not give in to a husband's controlling demands.

The following woman, who is 54 years old and eighty pounds overweight, says that her husband stopped being sexual right before their fifteenth wedding anniversary. They had started a new business, and he was working long hours and rarely home.

At first I thought he was just tired, but I had begun to gain weight at that point, too. I wasn't fat then, just a little overweight. I tried to seduce him, which he didn't react to, so I became angrier and angrier and that was when I started to eat and drink more and more.

Clearly, there may be underlying psychogenic factors surrounding obesity. As sex therapists Gerald Weeks and Nancy Gambescia state when writing about the phenomena of perceived body image and inhibited sexual desire: "The emphasis on appearance [can be] a red herring or a simple explanation for a deeper, unrecognized problem." June Reinisch says: "If a person gains that kind of weight, it can be a problem for some men. The question is: what's happening in her life and in their lives that it can occur? It really doesn't happen overnight, we can all agree. A woman doesn't gain ninety pounds in a year." When asked if she believed it to be a fear of intimacy, unexpressed anger, or hostility, Dr. Reinisch replied: "It could be [any or] all of those things or her unhappiness due to depression. The question is, when a woman starts to gain a lot of weight, what's going on in their relationship that they haven't dealt with together, as a couple?"

> I think his lack of sexual interest is one of the main reasons I had gained the weight. I didn't put on weight until after we stopped having sex. Looking back, I think it was my way of giving myself an excuse for his no longer wanting me. I gained forty pounds and have taken twenty off. **(Female, 30s)**

SOME MEN DON'T WANT THEIR WIVES TO LOSE WEIGHT

Most women aspire to be thin, but if they aren't, there are men who prefer it that way. Some men don't want a trophy wife because *they* want to be perceived as the prize. Others feel superior because they are thin as Jack Sprat, but their wives resemble his spouse. Although these men may pretend to encourage efforts to lose weight, they secretly hope for failure.

A man might say he wants his wife to lose weight, but in actuality be threatened by her doing so. A newly thin wife might expect her husband to be more sexual, especially if he has been saying he lost passion because of her weight gain. Stuart and Jacobson give an example of a man falsely blaming impotence on his wife's obesity, and then having to sadistically continue the charade to avoid the truth: "For years he refused to have sex with me, claiming that he only found slender women attractive. Believing this, I worked hard at losing weight, and actually got to three pounds under goal. But he still says I'm too fat. Currently he points to his secretary, who is 5'10" and weighs 115 pounds as a woman that he finds sexy." In their research, men were often depicted as cruel, comparing their spouses unfavorably to thinner actresses, acquaintances, or even former lovers. Many were accused of sabotaging attempts at weight loss by bringing home fattening foods or complaining about the expense of a health club membership. Some women even reported physical abuse as they were close to attaining their goal.

Other men are apprehensive that a slender wife might stray, or is getting thin for some other guy. They might think a newly attractive partner might demand more attention, complicating a life they find comfortable. Or they may simply dislike change.

AND SOME MEN WANT TO HELP

Of course, some husbands genuinely care about their wives and want them to lose weight for positive reasons; they just don't explain themselves effectively. Dr. Reinisch, who believes conversation should begin early, after a weight gain of about twenty pounds, suggests expressing concern without negativity. The husband might start by saying: "Honey, what's going on here? It's not that I'm losing my attraction for you, but something's wrong here where you are gaining so much weight. What's going on in your life? What can we do as a couple?" Sharing in a problem and its solution, rather than making it one-sided, is an effective tactic for any marital conflict.

Some men feel deeply rejected by their partner's weight gain and refusal to diet and exercise, believing that it is an indication that she just doesn't care if she's sexy anymore and therefore doesn't love him. Just as it seems illogical that one can stop being sexual for years, do nothing about it, and still demand fidelity from a mate, it seems equally illogical that one can gain a great deal of weight and adopt a less than healthy lifestyle and still expect to be desired with frequency and great passion. Both situations are possible, of course, but unrealistic, and tend to exist within the boundaries of religion and culture, not logic.

A BATTLE FOR CONTROL

My wife has never been a petite woman, but in college she was not nearly as heavy as she is now. In 1983, I asked her to marry me but asked that she promise to lose some of her extra weight. She agreed, so we got married. It took about two years for me to realize that she had no intention of losing weight. In fact, she started getting bigger. We began to fight about her weight but kept having sex. The fighting and growing lack of attraction on my part began to take its toll both in frequency and quality of the sex until I told her not to touch me anymore. We have not had sex in sixteen years. Her weight has gotten up to 350 pounds. She currently weighs around 260 pounds— she is 5′5″. (Male, 40s)

The man in the preceding quote married a woman who, in his opinion, needed to lose weight. Similar to the man quoted at the beginning of this chapter, he intended to turn her physically into the woman he desired, a plan that was doomed to fail, leaving him frustrated and in need of exerting power in some other way. His partner responded by not only refusing to lose weight but gaining more, checkmating their relationship at the expense of her health. With a current BMI of 43.3, she would be classified as morbidly obese. In a follow-up interview, we asked if there was any other reason the intimacy stopped. He replied:

There wasn't at first. In the beginning, weight was the only issue. However, after all these years I just don't feel an emotional connection with my wife anymore. At this point, even if she lost lots of weight, I don't think we could reconnect physically or emotionally. I'm not sure what will happen to us. I'm committed to getting my son through college; we are not in the best of shape financially so staying together will help. After that, I'm not sure.

When questioned about his wife's reaction, he answered:

There hasn't been much reaction. My wife has always been pretty tight-lipped about her feelings. She has said some things about it—that it hurt her when I refused to have sex with her. But, most of the past sixteen years she has barely acknowledged it.

When asked if he had any other sexual outlets, he said:

I was celibate for the first eleven of the sixteen years; since then I've had several affairs and a number of casual encounters. Besides getting just sex, I've gotten companionship, warmth, and intimacy.

He says his father-in-law is "harsh, judgmental, and overbearing—always on her about her weight. I really think staying fat is a way of her resisting his control of her."

Curiously, he blames her father, seemingly unaware of replicating the man's negative pattern. He takes no responsibility for his own bad behavior. His wife is staying in a relationship that is unpleasant but familiar, and it is possible that her lack of acknowledgment about sexual problems and obesity are a way of keeping some control, no matter how dangerous, over her life.

IS THERE SEX AFTER WEIGHT LOSS?

Thirty-five percent of the male respondents answered yes to the question "If a reason was weight gain, do you think you would have sex with your wife again if she lost weight?" Forty-two percent said they didn't know, and the rest (23%) answered they would not. The women were skeptical that weight loss would result in bringing sex back into the marriage. Although 47 percent said they were trying to lose weight, only 10 percent of the dieters were certain it would make any difference, 52 percent were uncertain, and 37 percent felt it wouldn't change a thing. They may be underestimating the positive physical and emotional results of weight loss on libido, their own as well as their partner's.

It is certainly possible to restore an active and exciting sex life once the pounds start to come off. Once a woman begins to diet seriously, her partner might be turned on by what he perceives as positive attention, and she might feel newly confident and sexual by the early success. Julian Slowinski cautions that the outcome might well be positive, but whether or not it is depends upon the rest of the relationship; June Reinisch said absolutely, if a couple deals with whatever the issues were that caused the weight gain in the first place. She adds that some women gain a lot of weight during pregnancy, and then keep it on, and that is something that the couple can beneficially work on together, as a team. If he doesn't need to lose weight, he can be her workout coach, changing his coaching venue from delivery room to gym. This puts him in a positive position where he is assisting with her health and well-being, at a time when she can really use the extra attention and support. And if and when she loses the weight, their sex lives will probably "come back with a roar."

We believe that if you are a significantly overweight woman married to a man who no longer desires intimacy, a sensible diet along with exercise is an excellent idea whether or not you think your weight gain contributed to the problem. Remember, you are losing weight for yourself, and not for him. However, aside from the previously mentioned health benefits, and they are numerous, the change in your appearance (and maybe even your sense of self-worth) may alter your husband's mood and trigger a rise in his levels of dopamine and norepinephrine.

eleven

MAYBE HE'S GAY? ASEXUAL?

I was kind of hoping that he was gay. I thought we could live together as friends and raise our kids. It would have been a relief that it wasn't about me and clear that there was nothing I could do about it. (Female, 40)

It's understandable that a woman might want to believe that the passionless man she's married to is, in actuality, not interested in her because he would prefer being intimate with other men. There would be nothing she could do; losing her anger or twenty pounds wouldn't mean a thing. It's not that he's just not that into her, he's just not that "into" her entire gender. It's in his genes, it's the way he was born, and she's in no way to blame for the lack of sex in their marriage. What a relief! And, oddly enough, it can be less painful for some women to believe that even if he's cheating, it's not with another woman.

However, most of our female respondents were realistic. They didn't think that their spouses were gay; in fact, 82 percent disagreed with the idea, and only 2 percent agreed with it. (Sixteen percent were neutral, which we interpret as uncertain.) Of the men, less than

1 percent identified as gay, and 4 percent as "neutral." About half the neutral men said they were bisexual.

It was once generally accepted that gay men (that is, men who have sex exclusively with other men) comprised about 4 percent of the total population in Western countries. The University of Chicago's seminal 1994 survey, however, looked at the question of sexual orientation differently. Focusing on 18- to 59-year-old men, it explored three different aspects of homosexuality: being sexually attracted to persons of the same gender, actually having sex with them, and self-identifying as gay. When phrased this way, 6 percent said they were attracted to other men, 5 percent claimed they had sex with another man at least once since they turned 18, but only 2.8 percent self-identified as homosexual.

It therefore becomes understandable that while only 2 percent of our female respondents are certain their spouses are gay and less than 1 percent of the males replied they were gay, many indicated uncertainty. Indeed, these men (and women) may be conflicted and confused. A 1990 study conducted by University of Chicago sociologist E. O. Laumann found that "3.9 percent of American men who had ever been married had sex with men in the previous five years." Laumann estimated that between 2 and 4 percent of American married women were either now, or had previously been, in marriages of "mixed orientation," and they may or may not have been aware of the situation.

However, it is also important to consider what a small percentage of the male population is, in actuality, homosexual, and that the Chicago studies were conducted in the 1990s. Much has happened since. Gay men are having commitment ceremonies and adopting children. Support for same-sex marriage has been tabulated as high as 40 percent in the overall population, and for college-aged people it is even more widely accepted. There is far less cause to be secretive about being gay; in most large American cities it's both accepted, and mainstream. Indeed, in America's twelve largest cities the gay population is estimated to be, on average, 9 percent. Few young men (at least in those large cities) have any realistic reason to keep their orientation private and to choose heterosexual marriage as the only way to have the "normal" family life of their dreams. (Some, however, may. As we write this, there are no openly gay senators or governors, which might be why Jim McGreevey, the former New Jersey governor who was blackmailed and "outed" by a former lover in 2004, made his clandestine lifestyle choice.)

Homosexuality is an unlikely—but possible—answer to the question of why men stop (or never start) having sex.

Like asexuality and extremely low testosterone, homosexuality is an unlikely—but possible—answer to the question of why men stop (or never start) having sex with their wives. Weeks and Gambescia state that although they have worked as therapists with such couples, the situation is rare. "These individuals may not wish to admit to themselves they are gay or admit it to the world." That is an important statement. A man may not realize that he is gay or may find the concept of admitting it to anyone, even himself, so negative that he remains closeted. Certain religious beliefs may make a gay lifestyle impossible to even contemplate.

BROKEBACK MARRIAGES

Men living in small towns, where homosexuality may not be as readily accepted, might be more likely to hide inside of "mixed-orientation" marriages. The popular 2005 film *Brokeback Mountain* told the tragic story of two small-town gay men torn between love for their wives, children, and each other. It put a sudden and strong spotlight on what are now called "brokeback marriages." Previously, Hollywood treated American gay male/straight female relationships frivolously. Take, for example, *In and Out,* a 1997 comedy in which Kevin Kline plays a beloved schoolteacher in a small Indiana town. In spite of his fondness for both elaborate window treatments and Barbra Streisand, not to mention the fact that he and his fiancée are in a sexless relationship, he does not realize he's gay. He can't even accept his orientation after being "outed" on national television, when a former student (now a famous actor), assumes that he's already "out" and thanks him for being the role model he channeled for his Academy Award–winning portrayal of a homosexual. However, by the end of the film it looks like a gay reporter (played by Tom Selleck) and Kline are going to live happily ever after. His former fiancée has no hard feelings, of course, and also finds true love. It is the ultimate feel-good, let's-all-be-open-minded-and-love-one-another fantasy. In 2004, Kline portrays Cole Porter in the fictionally fantasized biopic *Night and Day,* this time as a bisexual but happily married man, whose wife appears to be only mildly upset when he spends some nights away from home with beautiful young men. These types of films all have one thing in common: the guy is gay, the gal is straight, and no one gets hurt. *Brokeback Mountain* was an astonishing change, a grown-up look at mixed-orientation marriage from every perspective. And everyone got hurt.

Heterosexual by Necessity, Not Desire

A 47-year-old gay respondent, married for twenty-three years to a woman of the same age, used the words in this heading to describe the pain of living in a mixed orientation marriage. He discovered that he was attracted to other men when still in high school, but chose a straight lifestyle instead.

> I was raised in the 1960s and 1970s and this was still the climate. I was a victim of a society that said being gay is wrong, and being married and having a family is the only socially accepted thing to do.

He wrote that although he told his wife about having a homo-sexual affair two years after the wedding, they both pretended it never really happened until about twenty years later, when he fell in love with a man and was no longer able to make believe he was part of a "typical" American family. (At this point they had three children.) He describes his wife as reacting to the news with anger, hurt, shock, betrayal, and hatred, and is critical of her lack of understanding and support. She, quite likely, was devastated by the realization that what she wished away twenty years ago had always been just under the surface, and what she tried so hard to believe in as real was all a fantasy.

Trying to sift through the past and separate fact from fiction is one of the most difficult things for any victim of infidelity, and it is arguably even harder to do this when you learn your spouse is gay. All those wonderful memories of family vacations, holidays, and celebrations—was he actually always thinking of someone else? What about when we made love?

People can attempt to force themselves and their spouses to live life the way they want it to be, instead of the way it is. Work, children, and the daily routine allowed the woman referred to in the quote to keep reality hidden away for decades, and it would have stayed that way if her husband hadn't finally decided that he could no longer live a lie.

> I became unfocused and noncommunicative, and I cried four or five times a day for no reason. I hated myself for being gay, and I hated my wife for not seeing what suppressing the feelings was doing to me as a man, husband, and father.

He writes that he and his spouse are about to separate. He blames society, his wife, and himself for the last twenty-three years of his life and says that he is still torn apart by depression and guilt.

The Inauthentic Life

Jim McGreevey is the former New Jersey governor we mentioned earlier who was caught in an elaborate self-made web of deceit and lies that ended in his 2004 resignation and proclamation "I am a gay American." In his memoir, he describes the torment of pretending to be straight to get elected and the hubris of living parallel lives. His political career and second marriage were brought down by his gay lover, a former subordinate and campaign aide placed in a high-paying government job he was unqualified for. He blackmailed him when the love affair ended, resulting in McGreevey divorcing his second wife and moving in with another man.

We thought about him a lot, this attractive, ambitious, powerful politician in his late 40s, twice married with a child by each wife. He admitted being very sexually active with multiple male partners before he finally settled into the tumultuous affair that led to his downfall. Did his current wife suspect homosexuality? Did his former?

The human sex drive can be powerful enough to topple empires, and has. Lust can soon resemble, or turn into, love. And love may conquer, love may destroy, but it can rarely be wished away—which is why we tend to romanticize anyone who does so for a noble cause (Rick Blaine in *Casablanca*, for example).

But when libido is weak, sex becomes an afterthought at most, no more than an occasionally pleasant, but unnecessary, diversion.

OR MAYBE HE NEVER LIKED SEX TO BEGIN WITH

My husband has never enjoyed sex. A wonderful man in every sense of the word, but he cannot show the emotion of love and sex. He does not view porn—I wish he would. I am in very good shape, but you cannot force someone to have basic needs like physical intimacy if they don't. **(Female, 40s)**

Sex is almost always required for an intimate, romantic, long-term committed relationship. It looms large as a chief component of exclusivity and fidelity, its frequency considered a barometer of the state of the union. Any other kind of close relationship can be, and usually is, devoid of sex, which may be why lifelong friendships are more common than golden wedding anniversaries. Once sex enters the game, a complex set of biological and psychological elements change all the rules.

"Marry your best friend" is advice that manages to be both good and bad at the same time. You can, after all, love your best friend, look forward to his company, laugh at his jokes, and go on terrific vacations. You can be, like the old song goes, a mutual admiration society. But if, hypothetically, you suddenly *fall* in love, he is supposed to evolve sometime during the courtship into your sensitive, passionate lover. If he falls into the lower end of the libido scale, he may manage to do just that, for a little while. But when the novelty-fueled passion that comes at the beginning of a new sexual relationship diminishes (if that passion ever really begins) and your "lover" goes away, leaving behind your best friend and you, what happens to the marriage? What can be done if you end up with a friend instead of a husband? As one respondent who has chosen to settle for a lifetime of sublimation told us:

> After ten years of marriage, I've resigned myself to the fact it will always be this way. I realize I have two choices: leave or learn to live with it. An affair is out of the question—I love him too much and I believe in the sacredness of marriage. I have decided to live a completely celibate life—no sex, no porn, no masturbation, and no fantasies. I treat my wanting sex as if it were an addiction, which is difficult because I was/am a very sexual person. Somehow I've managed. I have put the energy into other things. I've lost weight, I'm no longer depressed,

and hubby and I have a very loving, albeit platonic relation-ship. He is a good father, a good provider, and a good friend. (Female, 32)

In our society, a man, especially, may be reluctant to reveal that he doesn't have a constant desire to have sex.

Others make the opposite choice, like this woman, also 32, who thinks that marriage to her childhood friend may soon end.

Our sex life died within the first six months of marriage. We've known each other our whole lives. I was actually his "first" back when we were kids. He says I am the love of his life, which I find hard to understand because he doesn't provide any "love." He is a good provider of everything else—but I always thought a marriage would have both elements. It's unfortunate; he really is an awesome person, and we are com-patible and close friends. But it can't last much longer. It makes me really unhappy.

There is a broad range of possible levels of sexual desire and the majority of men and women fall within it. Some people, however, fit into the category of those who have either a very high or low level of desire or none at all. Whether or not one's libido is below average can be difficult to assess in a culture that embraces the concept of sexual-ity in all things, including diet soda and mouthwash. When media and advertising represent a state of constant arousal as the norm, it may be embarrassing, even considered "abnormal," to not want a lot of sex. Thus, an individual with a low libido may cover it up, similar to a gay or lesbian of decades past. In our society, a man, especially, may be reluctant to reveal that he doesn't have a constant desire to have sex.

Conventional wisdom is that men have a stronger sex drive than women, and statistical data and clinical research seem to verify this. In a 1991 study, almost all the men (91%) but only half the women (52%) experienced sexual desire several times a week. A 1995 study concluded that men had more frequent and more varied sexual fantasies. A 2001 extensive review of the psychological literature surrounding the issue of gender differences in sexual motivation concluded that it was "indisputable," based on the "quantity, quality, diversity and convergence of the evidence," that men desire sex more than women; it went on to state: "We did not find a single study, on any of nearly a dozen different measures, that found women had a stronger sex drive than men." And in a 2006 online survey of long-term relationships implemented by *Elle* magazine and MSNBC, 66 percent of the almost thirty-nine thousand male respondents said they wanted more sex than their partner.

Many of the men that we have been discussing in this book may have average or even strong sex drives, but don't want to be intimate with their partners. The men we are discussing *here,* however, have below-average or low sex drives, and their wives have nothing to do with it. And then, there are men with a complete lack of sexual desire. Asexuality is rare, but it does exist.

ARE THERE *REALLY* MEN WITH LOW LIBIDOS?

He has no sex drive. Is he asexual and doesn't know it? (Female, 59)

HSDD, which stands for hypoactive (underactive) sexual desire disorder, is the term used when desire for sex, partnered or solitary, is infrequent. The American Psychiatric Association defines it like this: "A persistently reduced sexual drive or libido, not attributable to depression, where there is reduced desire, sexual activity, and sexual fantasy."

The APA also stipulates that in addition to depression, low libido cannot be diagnosed as HSDD if it is the result of a general medical condition (i.e., obesity or diabetes) or substance use (including prescriptive medication, alcohol, or street drugs). This suggests that if any or all of these conditions were resolved, libido would most likely be restored, but if it isn't, only then would HSDD be an acceptable diagnosis. Age and overall physical health are taken into account.

However, HSDD has also become an all-encompassing term used to describe individuals with significantly lower than average sexual desire, for any reason. Studies have shown it to be more prevalent in females (33%) than males (20%).

Trying to quantify the amount of sex an individual should want might seem foolhardy, as each of us is unique. It is, however, done all the time, by magazines, universities, and even the government. Remarkably, the statistics regarding frequency of intercourse for married couples seem to consistently fall, on average, between one and three times per week, declining with age. *Sex and the City* and other single-centric television shows notwithstanding, married people have more sex than singles, probably due to easy availability.

"Normal," when discussing sexual appetite, is a complex, delicate, and misleading term.

Since men appear to want sex more than women do, it would seem likely that a man suffering from HSDD is rare. It is not. Therapist Michele Weiner Davis states: "Based on my clinical observations and conversations with colleagues, low sexual desire in men is considerably more rampant than many people think." Therapists David Schnarch and Joseph LoPiccolo would agree; both say that of couples who see them for loss of desire, at least half the time it is the man who has stopped wanting intimacy in the marriage.

When HSDD is used as a catchall term for little or no sex, it may be the result of so many factors that it can be difficult to pinpoint the causative reasons. It may be psychological in origin, linked to anger, stress, or fear; physiological, caused by hormonal imbalances, such as a low level of testosterone; or the unintended result of medication for a wide variety of diseases including diabetes and vascular issues. Depression can result in a lack of desire, and, as we previously mentioned, so can antidepressants. It may be true HSDD and biological in origin, simply the way an individual functions; just as one man may have an unusually high sex drive, another may have one unusually low. And sometimes a man with a weak level of desire marries a female with a libido that falls into a range that is average or above, a situation perhaps masked in the early days of courtship when his passion was able to soar to a temporary high before it peaked and declined back to what is "normal" for him.

"Normal," when discussing sexual appetite, is a complex, delicate, and misleading term. It suggests there is something wrong, or abnormal, about a low libido, and there is not. Let us state again, there is a very wide range of normalcy when it comes to desire, and even that is fluid, changing with age, health, opportunity, partner, and state of mind. It can morph from quiet, occasional yearning to immense, wild, uncontrollable passion and back again. To quantify passion is to put a figure on the unique.

Problems arise when a couple's level of desire is disparate. When we discuss HSDD in this chapter, we are talking primarily about biological and hormonal issues, things beyond the sphere of anger, psychogenic wounds leading to fear of intimacy or even touch, religious-based causatives that inhibit deeply sexual feelings of any type deemed "wrong," or a simple lack of attraction. We are also eliminating those men who prefer, for whatever reason, solitary sex. That leaves us with men who rarely or never fantasize or desire partnered sex.

ASEXUALS HAVE OTHER THINGS
ON THEIR MINDS

It is difficult to imagine a man without fantasies of a sexual nature or history of solitary or partnered sex, and in fact such a man would be hard to find. Asexuality is a rare condition, and even rarer among men than women, but it does exist.

In 2004, researcher Anthony Bogaert published a national study on asexuality. One percent of adults self-identified as asexual, which is defined as having no attraction to males or females. Women are more likely to be asexual than men. A minority of both men and women (but more women) who said they were asexual reported that they were currently in long-term cohabiting or marital relationships.

It isn't sexy to be asexual; and some asexuals allege discrimination. Members of AVEN (Asexuality Visibility and Education) believe that the American Psychological Association should allow for four sexual preference possibilities instead of three, adding asexual to their current list of heterosexual, homosexual, and bisexual. The isolation asexuals once experienced has been alleviated somewhat by the Internet, where there are now support groups and websites. The AVEN site has a store that sells T-shirts with sayings like "Asexuality. It's not just for amoebas anymore," and, for those in partnered relationships, "I'm Asexual and So Is My Significant Other!" There is talk of "A-Pride."

Clearly, two people with no sexual desire at all can be happily married, as long as it's to each other. It is also clear that if an asexual marries someone with an average libido, whatever that may be, problems will arise that are likely to be insurmountable.

Having said that, such a tiny portion of the extremely small male asexual population marries, that it is very unlikely that this is the reason that a married man stops having sex. It can seem comforting to think that one's partner is asexual (the responsibility for the problem falls entirely on him, and at least there's no other person involved), but this is usually not the case—the odds are simply against it.

LESS THAN TEN TIMES A YEAR

> I believe my husband just has a low libido, but I was unaware of this when we got engaged. We pretty much stopped having sex about three months after moving in together, and four years ago we stopped completely. He has no interest in even finding out why he isn't interested. **(Female, 38)**

HSDD is usually quantified as wanting to make love ten times a year or less. It is possible that a man may be happy; healthy; free of stress, intimacy issues, and anger; not suffering from erectile dysfunction or on libido-reducing medication; not drug dependent or obese; not spending time watching online porn or engaging in other types of masturbatory fantasy; not having an affair, bisexual leaning toward gay, or gay; a good husband, father, in love and content with his life and wife; and still not want to have sex very often.

It's possible, but extremely unlikely, because HSDD is usually not a stand-alone issue. If you really believe that with your partner it is, and everything else in the relationship is fine, look a little harder, talk a little longer, and listen a lot closer. If you still are convinced it is not related to anything else, you have to decide how to deal with the fact that your partner loves you and finds you desirable; he just doesn't, or can't, show it in a sexual way. Unfortunately, he's in control, whether he wants to be or not. The person with lower desire always is. Many self-help books (and therapists we have interviewed over the years) suggest some type of compromise: he can watch you masturbate, or perform oral sex with no need for you to reciprocate. To be realistic, most men will be awkward about admitting their libido is so much lower than their partner's, and/or not interested in the servicing aspect. It may also be embarrassing for a woman to do these acts in front of a disinterested party. However, if he is willing and participates with love and enthusiasm, this might be an interim solution. Often, those who suffer from HSDD (as opposed to those who are asexual) find enjoyment in sex once they actually start doing it. They don't have the fantasies and general feelings of desire, but they can experience great pleasure once they start making love if they can allow themselves to get lost in the moment.

WHAT ABOUT LOW TESTOSTERONE?

The Massachusetts Male Aging Study assessed the sex drive and hormonal levels of 1,632 men between the ages of 40 and 70 years old. At each of three points in time during a fifteen-year period (1987–1989, 1995–1997, 2002–2004), the men were asked to complete self-administered questionnaires about the frequency of sexual thoughts, desires, and fantasies, and their level of testosterone was measured. At the start of the study, based on the questionnaires, 19 percent of the men were classified as low libido. This number increased as the subjects got older, 23 percent at the second time period, when 922 of the original men were still available, and 28 percent at the third, when 623 men remained. A team of scientists evaluated the data in the *Journal of Clinical Endocrinology and Metabolism*. They reported a statistical link between men's sex drives and testosterone levels, although the difference in levels of men self-reporting as high, average, or low was so small that they concluded: "The value of individual patient reports of reduced libido as indicators of low testosterone is open to question." In other words, if a man's sex drive is low, it may not be due to low testosterone. As we have discussed, there are multiple physiological and psychological reasons for a man not wanting to have partnered sex.

However, it is also possible that an abnormally low level of testosterone, a steroid hormone manufactured in the testes and in minuscule amounts, the adrenal glands, is the cause. In animal testing, males deprived of testosterone will not initiate or participate in sex with a willing partner, although they can achieve an erection if stimulated. The Massachusetts Male Aging Study estimated that there were about 2.4 million 40- to 69-year-old men in America with a testosterone deficiency. A blood test, usually administered in the morning because testosterone level is highest at that time, can attempt to determine if this is the case. The level is usually higher in autumn and can fluctuate with emotion and stress; therefore, the test is sometimes administered more than once. It is extremely difficult to achieve accuracy when measuring this hormone even with repeated testing, making the number of men with abnormally low testosterone difficult to estimate.

A man's level of testosterone peaks during adolescence and declines thereafter, dropping about 1 percent a year. Thus, the level is most likely to be lower than normal, and result in diminished sex drive, when a man is over the age of 60. (Some decline might be a good thing for the man's partner—he may focus more on foreplay and less on his own pleasure.) The range of testosterone considered "normal" is enormous—anything between 300 and 1200 nanograms per deciliter is sufficient. Although it is theoretically possible for levels to drop down so low that libido is diminished, it is unusual for this to actually happen, and it is therefore possible that testosterone may be administered unnecessarily. In a *New York Times* article dealing with middle age, loss of libido, and the "so-called syndrome called andropause," Dr. Richard A. Friedman states, "the vast majority of men who have these complaints [fatigue, loss of muscle mass, decreased libido] do not have testosterone levels in the deficient range. . . . In fact, many of these so-called testosterone deficient men actually have depression, alcohol problems, or other diseases that have gone undetected."

But for men accurately diagnosed with abnormally low levels of testosterone, medication can be life altering. There are a variety of treatments including pills, gels, patches, and injections. Increasing the hormone to normal levels can raise libido and enhance overall feeling of well-being. However, *these are not medications to be tinkered with in hopes of regaining youth or enhancing sexual prowess*—the side effects can be serious, and include increased risk of stroke, stimulation of undetected prostate cancer cells, and enlargement of the prostate. Your primary care physician will most likely recommend that you visit an endocrinologist if he believes treatment is necessary.

THE BELL CURVE

When we asked clinical psychologist Dr. Julian Slowinski about female respondents who claimed that everything was fine, except that their husbands just didn't want sex very often, he replied: "That's possible. You have to think of a bell curve. There will be guys over to one end that are highly sexual, and guys on the other who are fairly nonsexual. And so, it would make sense that if he is one of the guys on the low end of the curve, she would complain about not having sex. The ideal is for low-sex people to find each other, so they can end up with a loving companion-like relationship instead of a sexual one."

In that ideal world, people with (permanently) low libidos would find one another and live happily and platonically ever after. As we mentioned, the Internet is helping statistically small groups of people, like asexuals, connect. It may also give those people who do want sex, but not very often, a chance to discover one another. However, if you are currently in a marriage that is wonderful except that your partner is on the low end of the bell curve and the reason is nonhormonal, there are difficult decisions to be made.

We don't want to appear sanctimonious (this is a second marriage for both of us and we know that a time can come when letting go is

We believe in staying together if it is at all possible to do so—but not at all costs.

the only choice, and that it can lead to better things), but here's what we believe: in our hearts, we hope that your choice will be to stay together. There are no perfect relationships in this world. We feel that one based on trust, humor, love, caring, support, and friendship, with perhaps a little tender lovemaking mixed in now and then, is worth holding on to and protecting. We are also aware of the "easy for *you* to say" factor here. We said it at the beginning of this book—we believe in staying together if it is at all possible to do so. Not at all costs, not if there is something so unacceptable to one or both of you that staying together is no longer an option. Only you can decide what the breaking point is and if it has been reached.

It just bothers us to think that a marriage that is terrific in every other way would be discarded because one person happens to be born on the low end of the libido curve.

PART III

what couples are doing about it

twelve

SHOULD I STAY OR SHOULD I GO?

I am okay with this. We still kiss, hug, snuggle, and cuddle. That is what is important to me and him. **(Female, 57)**

The future of my marriage is not very bright. My husband is a wonderful man, but I just don't want a companion at this stage of my life. **(Female, 46)**

Here's another surprise: the overwhelming majority of our respondents are not divorced, and most of them don't seem to be thinking about it. Half of all marriages in America end; but only 10 percent of the men and 15 percent of the women who answered our survey are no longer married. That is not to say they are *happily* married, or that some are not considering breaking up in the future.

To be alone can be frightening or exciting—it all depends on one's point of view and stage of life. For some, any relationship is preferable to none. Children or financial issues may prevent separation or provide an excuse to stay, even if leaving is a better choice. Some were admittedly unhappy, "doing nothing," and resigned to a future of more of the same. But many respondents seemed satisfied in every room of the house except the bedroom. Perhaps they have made peace with the fact that their marriage is without passion but not without love, and that is considered to be fair exchange.

> I don't think we have a bad marriage. Sex is not the only thing we have. It would be better if we had it more, but I'm still happy. (Female, 28)

WHEN COUPLES CHOOSE TO PART

We found that ED, depression, anger, discovering a computer down-loaded with pornography, or even an affair was usually not reason enough to call the divorce lawyer.

Of that small population that *did* divorce, what were the reasons? The vast majority of the men said they were angry; they were also more likely to identify as bored, on medication, and depressed and to believe their spouses were unfaithful. They reported slightly less sexual dysfunction, perhaps indicating that they weren't as fearful of competing in the world of single men. Only 11 percent of those who had an affair divorced.

As for the women, it astonished us that less than half identifying their husbands as gay left their marriage. Sexual dysfunction was rarely a reason to separate; even those who reported that their part-ners had ED and refused to get help were unlikely to leave. Women who self-identified as having an affair were slightly more likely to di-vorce than those who remained faithful.

MEN AND WOMEN ON THE COUCH

Contrary to the conventional wisdom that women are more likely than men to seek psychiatric help, about the same percentages (30%)

of women as men entered therapy, either alone or together. Both were somewhat more likely to divorce than those who didn't seek counseling. It is possible that they did not stay with their therapist long enough, or that this was the wrong therapist for them, or that the therapist was incompetent. It may have been too little, too late. It is also feasible to imagine a therapist helping a couple separate with dignity, peace, and hope for the future.

FOR THE SAKE OF THE CHILDREN

Many couples put their own happiness in storage for the sake of their children. They may be noble—and they may be right. According to sociologist Paul Amato, an estimated 55–60 percent of children from divorced homes are not as happy as they used to be when their parents were together. However 40–45 percent are *more* content. Leaving a house filled with uncontrollable rage or simmering low-level anger can be a relief for children old enough to be aware of chronic tension. Many children from single-parent households thrive, although it should be mentioned that children of divorce have twice the emotional problems of children from two (biological) parent households. In 2000, almost 40 percent of America's children were living in a family other than one with their two biological parents.

Quite a few of our respondents said they were hanging in there just until their kids were old enough to leave the house. Of course, saying isn't doing. One 78-year-old man said he and his 76-year-old wife were "staying together for the sake of our married daughters and seven grandchildren." Children may provide an easy (or perhaps righteous) excuse to stay, while ignoring serious issues. Fear of being alone, loss of assets or financial support, familiarity, friends, and remembrance of things past are all valid considerations and cannot be ignored.

The following 41-year-old man says he is angry and depressed, and suffers from inhibited ejaculation, and that the rare times he is intimate with his wife, the sex is "boring." His youngest child is 4.

> On everything except sex, we're really close. Our views on reli-
> gion, money, and children are all similar. It's just this one area
> that we're really lacking in. Sometimes I think I'll split the sec-
> ond our youngest reaches 18, and other times I figure "why
> bother?"

This man is trying to convince himself that his marriage would be ideal if it weren't for the infrequent and "boring" sex. We doubt his wife would agree with this, especially since he takes no responsibility for their sexual problems.

He is, however, most likely speaking with bravado when he talks about "splitting" in fourteen years if he considers it worth the effort. This guy probably isn't going anywhere, unless his wife asks him to.

Others used their children as an excuse to sleepwalk through marriage, transforming their homes into prisons. They cross off days on their perpetual mental calendar, dreaming of the time they will be free at last. The following woman is an example of this. She is staying put until the children are grown.

> I don't think of myself as being married, I think of him as a good
> roommate. Our marriage should last about another two years
> until our youngest has graduated high school; I don't want to
> shake up his world too much while he's still living at home and
> in school. I'm also trying to increase my financial independence.
> (Female, 54)

In many of these situations, the children have become a convenient way for parents to fool themselves into believing they would be courageous enough to leave the marriage, if it weren't for the kids. It can be a way for a man suffering from sexual dysfunction to ignore his fear of being unable to satisfy a new partner. It can allow an angry woman, worn out by feeling undesirable and ignored, but unsure of being able to support herself, to avoid taking the risk.

Obviously, it is preferable for children to grow up in a loving two biological parent household. However, putting the children first is so clearly the "right thing to do" that the absence of love can be ignored, and self-righteousness can take the place of self-exploration. Without trying to understand *why* they are marking marital time, a couple may keep their marriage intact "until the children are grown" or even until the grandchildren are grown—but a life on hold is far from the ideal.

We encourage couples who are staying put "until" to analyze all the reasons why they are planning to divorce in the future. This should be done openly, honestly, and together. And without shifting responsibility to the kids.

> There are many things that we would throw away...
> If we were not afraid that others might pick them up.
> (Oscar Wilde)

Some women won't leave because they can't stand the thought of anyone else replacing them in their husband's world. The woman in the next quote told us she was unhappy in her marriage, enjoyed a good career, and had no children, but did not want to hand over her luxurious life to a younger woman.

> Last year my husband made partner and the $$$ are really flowing in—I'll be damned if I'll leave him when we have everything. Also realizing a young twentysomething would be close by to bag him (we are both 36 now).

What unfortunate reasons to stay in a marriage—the fear that someone else may snag the guy you don't want, and that at 36 you're too old to "bag" another successful man. This woman wrote that she and her husband have been unfaithful to each other, and she is unhappy. Nevertheless, she is willing to put up with anything. We live in a society where many people consider a woman married to a big earner a success, even if the marriage is without intimacy and she's bringing home the "$$$," too. If she thinks she may never hook as big a fish again, that becomes reason enough for her to remain unhappily married. For others, just the status of being married is the thing that can't be tossed away, because they are afraid someone else will soon attach themselves to their ex, and there is too much risk in not having a readily available escort, or being alone on a Saturday night, or, most of all, never finding a replacement. The concept of "I'd rather be married than single no matter the emotional price" seems archaic, but for some, it's a way of life. The respondent we just quoted was honest enough to say something we suspect many others feel, but might not even want to admit to themselves.

The inability to discard a mate might also be attributed to this fear: if a women's spouse has stopped being sexual with her, she may want to prevent him from becoming attached to, and therefore intimate, with somebody new, because if that were to happen she would have to face the unfortunate truth that she just wasn't attractive to him, after all.

THE WISDOM TO KNOW THE DIFFERENCE

Physical and emotional abuse, drug addiction or alcoholism—any of these, without remorse and commitment to change, are reasons to consider divorce. It would be comforting to know that most people eventually get the courage to leave such relationships, wondering how they could have stayed so long. It is not possible, however, to know if this is really true. Reliable studies are rare since it is extremely difficult to quantify abuse. In addition, it is likely to be underreported or falsely reported.

Our survey and research focuses on marriages without passion, due to personal insecurities and private demons—a fear of intimacy, say, or a struggle with impotence. However, a man may stop having sex for reasons that stem from the extreme edges of the norm, either his partner's or his own. When this occurs, sometimes respect (and self-respect) are gone as well, resulting in behavior that is intolerable. The majority of our respondents did not seem willing to live with an addict, eventually coming to the realization that when there is substance abuse or other kinds of long-term, untreated addiction, and the situation shows no signs of improving, it is time to go.

> She got hooked on gambling. It was more important than the kids, me, or anything else. (Male, 66, divorced after fifteen years of marriage)

> The future of the marriage is not good. My wife is seeing a therapist, but she still drinks heavily and that is a big reason we don't have sex. (Male, 58, separated after twenty-three years of marriage)

Unlike the two men we just quoted, others decide to stay in a miserable situation. The woman quoted next is clinging to her "soul mate" in spite of what appears to be an extremely bleak partnership with a man who is doing nothing to change. She describes her husband as angry, depressed, and on libido-lowering medication. He suffers from ED, premature ejaculation, and inhibited orgasm, which is not surprising when she reveals his lifestyle. He stopped having sex with her in the first year of marriage.

> He drinks Jim Beam to excess every day, smokes marijuana, and ingests cocaine. He runs away from home for days at a time. This is the third marriage for us both and I can honestly say that I love him with all my heart. I truly believed that I had found my soul mate. Nothing prepared me for the domestic abuse, the cruelty, or the disappointment. I am considering divorce. (Female, 49)

Since it is clear that this woman isn't staying married for religious reasons, and has gotten divorced twice before, it is puzzling that she is just "considering" divorce from a man she describes as cruel and abusive. Clearly she doesn't do well at choosing husbands and should explore, perhaps with the support of a therapist or member of the clergy, why she is making such poor choices, and why she can write that she still loves a monster "with all my heart."

The next woman we quote finally did leave, although it took extreme physical abuse to get her to do so. She describes a marriage that is intolerable in almost every way—and yet she stayed in it for more than ten years.

> We separated because of the escalating violence from him. I did begin to have affairs in the last few months; it was my way to prove to myself men still found me desirable. I believed he had someone long before my affairs . . . I found pictures . . . and he came home later and later as time passed. (Female, 49)

When a 66-year-old man, divorced after a twenty-five-year marriage, told us: "She was an alcoholic and was in love with the bottle," we asked him what he would have done differently, if he could do it all over again. He simply answered: "Learn the Serenity Prayer and follow its advice."

The Serenity Prayer is attributed to theologian Dr. Reinhold Niebuhr, and it is beautiful in its simplicity—*God grant me the serenity/To accept the things I cannot change/Courage to change the things I can/And wisdom to know the difference*. This obvious but often overlooked truth that we have no control over so many things, including the past and a spouse who refuses to stop behaving badly, can be a revelation. It took this man more than twenty years to realize he had no power over his wife's alcoholism, but he did have control over his own life, and the courage to finally change it.

thirteen

WHAT WOMEN ARE DOING ABOUT IT

It seems indisputable that whoever has the lowest level of desire controls the frequency of sex in a partnered relationship. If that happens to be the man, many women are dealing with the situation by turning to an additional partner. Twenty-four percent of the women said that they began having an affair *after* their husbands stopped being sexual. This number is considerably higher than the one published by the University of Chicago's National Opinion Research Center (11.3%), or the 2006 Elle Magazine/MSNBC survey (14%), but they do not specify women in sexless marriages. Only 9 percent of our female respondents said that they were having an affair *before* their husbands stopped being passionate. It is interesting to note that although the men who choose to be nonsexual within their marriage are not having significantly more affairs than the national average, their wives are.

Can a person who is one-half of an equal partnership make a unilateral decision to be celibate and expect fidelity?

A 53-year-old woman, married for twenty-three years, put it like this:

> I am having a real affair, not online. My husband hasn't touched me in fifteen years. I gained thirty pounds with my pregnancy in 1984 and have taken it off and put it back on over the years. When I am slimmer, he doesn't seem any more interested in sex, but I am.

A 47-year-old woman whose husband stopped being intimate with her because he suffered from impotence said this about her new lover:

> The person I'm having an affair with also has ED, and we have found all sorts of ways to pleasure each other sexually.

This woman, 52, has been married to her 54-year-old husband for thirty years. He stopped being sexual with her eight years ago and suffers from ED. She told us about her lover:

> I got more out of this affair than I ever expected both physically and emotionally. One really important thing for me was that it pushed me to reexamine my marriage and made me realize that it is over.

A 43-year-old woman remarked:

> I needed the affairs to let me know what I was capable of. At the time, I wasn't feeling very feminine or very womanly. I think if I didn't have the affairs, I would have continued to feel that way about myself. The affairs also helped me to have the confidence to get divorced.

Can a person who is one-half of an equal partnership make a unilateral decision to be celibate and expect fidelity? Does the partner who is being refused sexual (and perhaps emotional) contact have the right to secretly seek it elsewhere?

Numerous tragedies and sad songs have been written about women crossing over to the cheatin' side of town. Like many of the female respondents to this survey, their reasons for going there are as likely to be unfulfilled emotional needs as physical ones. Feeling *anything* resembling affection might be intoxicating, after long periods of being turned down by the man who is supposed to love you. The hormones that accompany a new sexual relationship can give a renewed sense of self-worth, and a visit back to a time of feeling desirable and adored. Not to mention terrific sex.

Some of the women said that their affair was a catalyst for divorce. That is understandable; the fears of leaving a marriage and facing life alone may disappear when there are other options. Even if they don't expect to begin a new life with their lover, a happy relationship sometime in the future seems suddenly possible.

Few things in life are more painful than betrayal by a loved one, as these men will probably discover. Some of the infidelity reported in our survey might have been avoided if the couples were open and honest about their problems from the start. Talking about difficult things, such as impotence or lack of intimacy is uncomfortable and unpleasant—not a conversation anyone wants to have. It is, however, infinitely superior to talking about infidelity.

DO WOMEN WHO REMAIN FAITHFUL CARE ABOUT SEX?

Oh boy, do they. Our respondents were a lusty group. Fifty-six percent self-identified as intensely or very sexual; another 27 percent said they thought they were average. Less than 4 percent felt they just weren't sexual at all. A 32-year-old woman who believes her marriage wonderful in every other way, said:

Excuse me? Are my husband and I freaks of nature? I have so much sexuality to give someone, and the man I love doesn't want it.

The majority, of course, said that they pleasure themselves—74 percent the old-fashioned way (that would be without a computer), and another 10 percent online. Less than 4 percent, however, said they visited online chat rooms for stimulation.

SOME TRIED THERAPY, TOGETHER OR ALONE

He said he would rather lose me and our daughter than go into counseling. **(Female, 35)**

Forty-four percent of the respondents said that they tried, unsuccessfully, to get their husbands into therapy. "He's just not a therapy kind of guy," said one woman, echoing many. Thirty percent of the women said they went into therapy alone.

Sadly, often couples begin therapy at the end of the road, when it is just too late.

Clinical psychologist Joseph LoPiccolo believes that "Most men are not comfortable with going to psychotherapy for any life problem, and this is especially true when the problem is a sexual one. I have stated this as 'Men who have a low drive for sex have an even lower drive for sex therapy'!"

Only 28 percent of respondents were successful in getting their spouse into counseling, and many claimed it was ineffective. (Please realize that if it *was* effective, they probably would no longer have a sexless marriage and wouldn't be answering our survey.)

Sadly, often couples begin therapy at the end of the road, when it is just too late. Sometimes neither person really wants to improve the situation; they just want their personal complaints validated, and when that doesn't happen, one or both turn away.

> We went but it was a joke. The female therapist was thoroughly charmed by him. When we got home, he said nothing was going to change. The therapist decided he was perfect and decided to blame the whole thing on my job. Never mind that he has a job that keeps him on the road at least half the time, too. (Female, 35)

It is more likely that the therapist didn't agree with everything the female patient said than decide that her husband was "charming" and "perfect." However, that's what the woman heard, and maybe her partner did, too, and it became a convenient excuse for them to stop therapy before it began.

CAN THERAPY HELP?

There are times when trying to work things out together, no matter how respectfully or honestly, doesn't work. And there are times when self-analysis doesn't give compelling solutions, either. If this is the case, there is no shame in needing someone else to talk to.

We suggest that the low-libido partner begin by visiting his primary care physician. He should bring a list of any medications he is taking. Any illness that might be causing an inability to get an erection, or inhibit orgasm, should be discussed. Lifestyle choices, such as excessive drinking, recreational drug use, smoking, and diet should be revealed as well. *Remember, it is necessary to be brutally honest about the sexual problems.* If the primary care physician suspects urogenital issues, he will probably refer the patient to a urologist.

Now, let's talk about therapy. As we have stated throughout this book, loss of libido is rarely a stand-alone problem, and therefore it is often best solved with an integrative approach. For example, a man may have success with a PDE5 inhibitor, but his wife may feel resentment for all the years he refused to get help. Is she now, perhaps, too old to easily become pregnant, and furious because she always wanted children? Suppressed thoughts on either side can crush desire. So can overt anger. Counseling may be helpful, by allowing a trained neutral third party to mediate expressed feelings and to reveal unspoken ones. Therapy can also help couples deal with the difficult issues of abuse, guilt, shame, and negative body image.

We caution you, however, to choose your therapist with care. (You can get referrals from your family physician, urologist, or from the APA website.)When you have some names, do your homework. You can't ask for references, but you can certainly ask for credentials. Be certain that the therapist's degrees are from well-established accredited universities. It is simple to further check credentials online. This is not to suggest that a therapist is necessarily better because he or she went to one school instead of another. But when you don't know a person's ability, and that person has the job of helping you save your marriage, credentials provide a shortcut to making a wise choice. It is extremely important to remember this: *if you are going for couple's therapy, make sure that the counselor has specific training in that area; it is probably the most difficult therapy to administer well.* That's because it becomes a very crowded room—the couple, of course, along with the attitudes they learned from their respective families. Before you commit to an appointment, speak to the therapist briefly by phone to describe your issue. If possible, see more than one before you make a final decision. If this is couple's therapy, make sure you both feel comfortable and agree with the choice.

Many marriages have been helped by couple's therapy. It can be very beneficial, but it has to be with a good therapist, embraced by all concerned, and committed to for a reasonable period of time.

How long should therapy last? Psychoanalyst Owen Renik says you should feel relief from some of your problems not long after beginning treatment. As he told the *New York Times,* "This idea that you have to wait around for a long time for the fruit to drop from the tree is nonsense. If you don't see progress soon, you should move on. If you don't see progress with the *next* person, fine; you may conclude that the process may take a little longer than expected." We concur. Marriage is supposed to last until death do you part; therapy isn't.

IN SPITE OF IT ALL, MOST STAYED TOGETHER

Of the aggregate women, 24 percent were having an affair *after* their husbands stopped being sexual and another 39 percent were thinking about it; of the men, 27 percent were having an affair *after* they stopped being sexual with their wives and 42 percent were considering it. Thinking isn't doing. Men and women in highly sexual marriages might also "think about" having an affair. Many people mentally try on other partners, only to reject the fantasy in favor of the marriage. But still, 63 percent of the women and 69 percent of the men were either having sex with someone other than their spouses, or seriously thinking about it. And they were staying together.

> I think there are a lot of women out there in the same situation and they stay because that's all they know after being with someone after so many years. (Female, 43)

Those who chose to stay did so for religious or spiritual beliefs, the children, out of fear of being alone or never finding someone better, economic pressure, or inertia. Many, however, did so out of love. They wanted an erotic life and they missed being sexual, but they seemed to feel, deep in their souls, that if they had to take their husband as best friend instead of lover, that was all right.

fourteen

AND IN THE END . . .

Were Lennon and McCartney right that the love you take is equal to the love you make? What if you are the only one who wants to take or make love?

There are no easy answers, and much of our impatience with self-help books is that they try to provide them. The problem with the self-help formulas is they have to work for more than just the self. You may be willing to reignite your sex life, but if your partner isn't, is it really all that helpful?

Over the years we have interviewed hundreds of sex therapists and marriage counselors and have heard all of the tried and not-so-true formulas for keeping sex hot in a long-term relationship. We wish we had a dollar for every time someone has suggested making love in a different room.

WE COULD NOT HAVE SAID IT BETTER

We are grateful to all the experts who have given us the benefit of their wisdom. But often, the best advice comes from those who are in the midst of this vexing and often painful situation.

What this next woman says certainly sums up best what we believe: you've got to talk to each other and, just as important, really listen. After all, there are just so many sexual positions, sexy lingerie, and bubble baths one can do, wear, or take. Ultimately, you have to face each other and break down the barriers between you and real intimacy.

I think that couples need to be able to talk about issues in marriage and sex in order to maintain emotional and physical intimacy. Some people come from families that never talked things over. This creates an almost insurmountable barrier and eventual boredom. Without new ideas, all you have left is repetition of roles previously played out. **(Female, 51)**

And we liked what the woman in the next quote said about agreeing to have what she and her husband call "our time." Setting aside some time every week to talk, or to connect physically with or without a sexual encounter, is a wonderful way to keep a relationship fresh.

Last month I finally got up the courage to discuss my feelings with him. He agreed to set aside time every week just for "our time." No TV or other distractions. It's time for us to talk or for sex. We're both working on losing weight. I'm working harder to please him in bed, hoping to get him more excited when anticipating "our time." I'm also trying to add some spice to "our time." **(Female, 43)**

Some people responded to our survey by telling us that they had a great sex life and marriage and wanted to tell us how they did it. The following man and his wife are both 66 and have been married for forty-nine years. Although perhaps not as frequent as it once was, sex is still an important part of their lives.

I think that sex has always been a strong bond in our marriage, so since we both enjoyed it so much we have just always taken the time to keep it interesting, exciting, and we have reinvented our sex life many times over. We still keep a romantic atmosphere in our bedroom, which is protected by both of us; we have a date night that we started when our children were at home, and we still practice even more now, and we work from a philosophy we discovered twenty years ago . . . smooch daily, date weekly, escape monthly, and vacation quarterly, and this has taken us on some really nice trips and exciting times together. We are always planning for the next escape or vacation, which we talk about often and that helps build the excitement.

We think this is a wonderful prescription, because they are working hard to stay connected on a variety of levels. The "romantic atmosphere" in their bedroom indicates that they are both committed to keeping intimacy alive; and the way they have instinctively evolved and changed their sex life over time has helped keep things exciting. Their weekly dates suggest that they still have a great time together, and a lot to talk about. The vacations, of course, add even more newness and anticipation.

In a similar vein, this 68-year-old man told us how he and his wife keep sex alive in their marriage of forty-three years:

It is less the physical attractiveness and more the emotional love and caring. We have so many shared values and common interests. We have made a great life for ourselves and occasionally sex is a part of it.

By "occasionally," he means six times a month. He says he compliments his wife every day and that he thinks she's beautiful. He told us: "I love my wife."

We were so grateful to all of our respondents, and especially to those who shared their formulas for happiness. How simple this man makes it seem: love, respect, and support each other, know that you are still attractive even if you are no longer twenty-five years old, and value the life you've shared together so much you work hard at protecting it. And tell that to each other every day.

THREE THINGS WORTH REMEMBERING

Clearly a lot of couples are not having sex because of ED. We've written extensively about the various prescriptive drugs on the market that work pretty consistently and safely—not for everybody, but for many. *If you're a man, and shame and embarrassment are stopping you from going to the doctor—get over it, and if you're a woman who feels threatened by your husband's need for a pill to get an erection—same advice.*

This brings us to our next point. *Please, if you haven't done so already, broaden your definition of sex.* Oral sex, mutual masturbation, touching, fondling—intimately connecting to each other with love fits our description. If intercourse is a problem for any reason, do something else.

One last piece of advice: *listen and listen carefully to what your spouse is saying.* It's one thing to talk about your problems (and we realize even that is not easy for some people). But truly listening with an open heart and mind to the pain, suffering, and desires of your mate takes effort and commitment. We often sensed that people weren't communicating their feelings honestly. But we feel even stronger that people aren't really listening to one another honestly. Nothing in our survey results illustrates our point better than this: 66 percent of the women agreed with the statement "He lost interest and I don't know why," but only 28 percent of the men agreed with the statement "*I lost interest and I don't know why.*" Either the men aren't talking, or the women aren't listening. The people in our survey are not married to each other, but we can't help but believe that on these key issues couples are not speaking up. So many seem to be living in a parallel marriage—they're in it together, and for the long haul, but they're not connecting physically or emotionally. It takes courage to truly connect with each other. It's hard to say what's really in your heart, and often difficult to hear your partner's strongest desires and fears. But we guarantee it's worthwhile.

We can't give you an absolute formula of how to do this—no one can. Every couple has a unique dynamic. But *you have to talk to each other,* and when you do, before you start, first pledge that you will respect each other's feelings and be nonjudgmental. You are trying to solve a problem, not prove you're right. And the problem belongs to you both—it is most definitely a "we" situation. Forget blame, and be willing to take responsibility. This may seem simplistic, but pay attention to your spouse—don't just wait for an opening to jump in and prove your point. *You have to listen, too.* There are probably a lot of built-up resentments and frustrations, or serious, painful issues like impotence and boredom to be dealt with. And don't expect to solve everything in one conversation. It will probably take a lot of talking, and listening, and that's a good thing. We truly believe that the majority of couples aren't really that far apart; they just have to communicate and do so with empathy.

WHEN *SHE* SAYS "NOT TONIGHT, DEAR, AND NOT TOMORROW NIGHT, EITHER"

After being told *NO!* 97 percent of the time, I finally decided to stop beating my head against the wall. I realized that never asking to have sex meant never being rejected again, so I stopped asking. I'm disappointed, but it sure beats begging and getting turned down all but once a month. (Male, 48)

We have said that a sexless marriage is rarely the result of only one partner's behavior, even if it looks that way on the surface. Putting aside those who go to extremes, the substance abusers who won't quit, the unfaithful without remorse—there are few if any marital problems that exist in a vacuum. Although the man that we just quoted says that not having sex is the choice of his 45-year-old wife and not him, he also told us that he suffers from erectile dysfunction. It is possible, therefore, that his wife of twenty-four years felt so rejected by his inability to get an erection that it was simply easier for her to turn him down. She may also be having some perimenopausal issues, such as vaginal dryness and/or painful intercourse. But they don't seem to be talking about any of this. Like so many men suffering from impotence, the blame has shifted and the problem remains unsolved.

> *A sexless marriage is rarely the result of only one partner's behavior, even if it looks that way on the surface.*

After years of being rejected sexually, I got tired of hearing no so I stopped asking. By the time my wife decided to initiate I was too angry and frustrated to say yes. It's easier to turn my sexuality off entirely than to subject it to being abused by my wife. (Male, 50s)

We mentioned earlier that the low-desire person in a sexless marriage is as likely to be the woman as the man. We decided to investigate the issue from the male perspective because we could find so little literature on the subject—the "problem" was usually considered to be caused by the woman. But as we read the responses of thousands of people generously willing to share time and intimate details with us—all the men and women who answered our survey because they believed that the first one to implement the no-sex, we're-married policy was the guy—we came to realize that the low-libido tag can usually be pinned on either partner first, almost at random, and "who started it" is unimportant. A middle-aged male may retreat because of impotence, his wife because of vaginal dryness, he visits an online porn site, she finds out, and then anger and rejection spiral everything out of control. A young man may prefer, early on, the no-risk, no-commitment approach to sexuality that only the Internet can provide; this may infuriate his wife and cause her to be constantly critical, and all hope of intimacy, which perhaps they both feared in the first place, flies out the bedroom door. Wife and husband may be bored, distressed that the passion they once readily enjoyed seems to elude them now, but neither is willing to do anything to recapture even a small portion of that early excitement. But which came first? Anger builds, resentment escalates, and passion fades. So which one is the "guilty" party? Who was careless enough to be the first one to lose their libido? It doesn't matter; the only thing that does is ending the constant shifting of blame. Take responsibility, talk openly and honestly, and listen, really listen to your partner with respect and love.

appendix

Methodology

We used thirteen websites to solicit participants for our survey, requesting people who self-identified as being in a sexless marriage either now or in the past where the man was the one to end the intimacy to respond. The majority of respondents came from www.thirdage.com. Other sites that provided a lot of participants included www.ivillage.com/mismatchedlibidos, various regional sites attached to the Man Kind Project (a men's personal growth organization), and topic-related sites from AOL, Yahoo!, and Google. This is not a scientific sampling of the general population, and self-reporting and volunteering surveys may attract a skewed sample.

More than four thousand people anonymously participated in our survey, 33 percent male and 67 percent female. Many agreed to follow-up online interviews for either additional information or clarification. The male mean age is 55, and mean years married is twenty-three. The female mean age is 48, and mean years married is fifteen.

The following demographics refer to all respondents.

Level of Education

High School	22%
College	54%
Grad School	23%

Annual Family Income in U.S. Dollars (thousands)

25–50	5%
51–75	20%
76–100	23%
101–200	22%
Above 200	6%

Country of Residence

United States	87%
Canada	5%
Europe	2%
Asia	2%
Australia and New Zealand	2%
Mexico	<1%
Central or South America	<1%
Africa	<1%

Religion

Protestant	34%
Catholic	23%
Other	21%
None	16%
Jewish	4%

Muslim	1%
Atheist	1%

After responding to the above, the survey branched by gender.

MEN'S SURVEY

When did you stop having sex with your wife?

1. Before we got married
2. On the honeymoon
3. First year of marriage
4. After the first year of marriage

The following are possible reasons you stopped having sex with your wife. For each statement, select an answer that corresponds with how important that reason is to you. (Note: We used a Likert scale with options: strongly agree, agree, neutral, disagree, and strongly disagree.)

I no longer find her physically attractive.
She has gained a significant amount of weight.
I am angry at her.
I am depressed.
She is depressed.
She isn't sexually adventurous enough for me.
She doesn't seem to enjoy sex.
I'm bored.
I lost interest and don't know why.
I am interested in sex with other people, but not my wife.
I suffer from erectile dysfunction.
I suffer from premature ejaculation.
I have difficulty achieving an orgasm.

I am on medication that lowered my libido.

I am/was having an affair.

She is/was having an affair.

I don't have the time.

I'm too tired.

I am gay.

I prefer to watch pornography online and masturbate.

I prefer to masturbate but not online.

I wasn't interested in sex to begin with.

If a reason was weight gain, do you think you would have sex with your wife again if she lost weight? (Yes, I don't know, No)

The Following Questions Were Answered by Yes or No, Unless Otherwise Noted

Did you have an affair after you stopped having sex with your wife?

Are you thinking about having an affair?

Did you go into counseling together?

Did you ask her to go into counseling and she refused?

Did you go to a therapist alone?

Do you watch online pornography? (Open-ended question: If yes, how many hours per week?)

Do you watch adult videos? (Open-ended question: If yes, how many hours per week?)

Did you separate after you stopped having sex?

Did you divorce?

Open-Ended Questions

What is your age?

What is your spouse's age?

How many years have you been married?

How many times did you have sex last year with your wife?

Please tell us what year of your marriage you stopped having sex with your wife. For example, year 5.

How many times did you have sex with your wife last year?

If there are other reasons, please explain.

Can you briefly describe what you mean? For example, if you find her physically unattractive, why? How has she changed? Or if you are angry at her, why? What are the issues?

What do you think the future of your marriage is?

If you could do things over again, what, if anything, would you do differently?

Is there anything you'd like to add?

WOMEN'S SURVEY

When did your husband stop having sex with you?

1. Before we got married
2. On the honeymoon
3. First year of marriage
4. After the first year of marriage

The following are possible reasons your husband stopped having sex with you. For each statement, select an answer that corresponds with how important you think that reason is. (Note: We used a Likert scale with options: strongly agree, agree, neutral, disagree, and strongly disagree.)

He no longer finds me physically attractive.

I have gained a significant amount of weight.

He is angry at me.

He is depressed.

I am depressed.

I am not sexually adventurous enough for him.

I don't seem to enjoy sex.

He's bored.

He lost interest and I don't know why.

He is interested in sex with other people but not with me.

He suffers from erectile dysfunction (impotence).

He suffers from premature ejaculation.

He has difficulty achieving orgasm.

He is on medication that lowered his libido.

He prefers to watch online pornography and masturbate.

He prefers to masturbate but not while online.

I am/was having an affair.

He is/was having an affair.

He doesn't have the time.

He wasn't interested in sex to begin with.

He is too tired.

He is gay.

How sexual do you feel at this point in your life? (Intensely, Very, Average, A little, Not at all)

The Following Were Answered by Yes or No, Unless Otherwise Noted

I masturbate, but not online.

I masturbate using online pornography.

I masturbate using chat rooms.

I am having/have had an affair.

I am having/have had multiple affairs.

I am thinking about having an affair.

Does your husband watch online pornography? (Open-ended
   question: If yes, how many hours per week?)
Does he watch adult videos? (Open-ended question: If yes, how
   many hours per week?)
If he suffers from erectile dysfunction (impotence), did he seek
   medical help?
If a reason was weight gain, do you think he would have sex with
   you again if you lost weight? (Yes, I don't know, No)
I am doing nothing.
I am trying to lose weight. (Yes, No, Not applicable)
Have you gone to counseling together for marital issues?
If no, did you ask him to go into counseling and he refused?
Did you go into therapy alone?
Did you separate after you stopped having sex?
Did you divorce?

Open-Ended Questions

Which year of your marriage did your husband stop having sex
   with you? For example, year 5?
How many times did you have sex with your husband last year?
If there are other reasons for not having sex, please explain.
Can you briefly describe the situation? For example, if you think
   he finds you physically unattractive, why? How have you
   changed? Or if you think he is angry at you, why? What are
   the issues?
What do you think the future is for your marriage?
If you could do things over again, what, if anything, would you do
   differently?
Is there anything you'd like to add?

notes

INTRODUCTION

4   *sex fewer than ten times per year*: Deveny, Kathleen. We're not in the mood. *Newsweek*, June 30, 2003. Having sex no more than ten times per year is what is considered by clinical sex therapists to be a "sexless" marriage, although many couples have less physical contact or none at all.

4   *lack of desire is recognized as the most common sexual problem in America*: Weeks, Gerald R., & Gambescia, Nancy. (2002). *Hypoactive sexual desire*. New York: W.W. Norton & Company, p. ix; also in Laumann, Park, and Rosen. (1999). United States Health and Social Life Survey.

4   *David Schnarch*: Schnarch, David. (2002). *Resurrecting sex*. New York: Quill, p. 16.

5   *Cathryn G. Pridal and Joseph LoPiccolo*: Pridal, Cathryn G., & LoPiccolo, Joseph. (2000). Multielemental treatment of desire disorders. In Leiblum, S. R., & Rosen, R. C. (Eds.), *Principles and practice of sex therapy* (3rd ed., pp. 57–81). New York: Guilford Press.

5   *we are referring to any long-term committed relationship*: For the first time, at 49.7 percent of total, and down from 52 percent only five years ago, married couples are a minority of American households, and those living unmarried, with partners, is increasing. Roberts, Sam. To be married means to be outnumbered. *New York Times*: October 15, 2006; Nearly half of Americans in their 30s and 40s have cohabited. Roberts, Sam. The shelf life of bliss. *New York Times*, July 1, 2007.

ONE. WHEN MEN STOP HAVING SEX

13   *"in the vast amount of couples consulting me about desire complaints it's the women who want more and the man who always has a headache"*: Zilbergeld,

Bernie. (1999). *The new male sexuality*. Revised Edition. New York: Bantam Books, p. 350.

16 *Drs. Max and Della Fitzgerald are clinical sex therapists:* Interview with the authors, July 24, 2006. All subsequent references to Dr. Max Fitzgerald and/ or Dr. Della Fitzgerald result from this interview.

17 *Dr. Helen Fisher, a research professor of anthropology at Rutgers University:* Interview with the authors, July 31, 2006. All subsequent references to Dr. Fisher result from this interview.

18 *Clinical psychologist and sex therapist David Schnarch:* Schnarch, David. *Passionate marriage*. (1997). New York. W.W. Norton, p.151.

26 *Hypoactive sexual desire disorder:* American Psychiatric Association. (2000). *Diagnostic and statistical manual of mental disorders* (4th ed.) (DSM-IV).

28 *A Newsweek cover…photographs an attractive heterosexual couple in bed:* Deveny, Kathleen. We're not in the mood. *Newsweek*. June 30, 2003.

TWO. WHY WOMEN THINK THEIR HUSBANDS STOP HAVING SEX

37 *American physicians wrote 118 million prescriptions for antidepressants in 2005:* Cohen, Elizabeth. CDC: Antidepressants most prescribed drug in U.S. *CNN.com.* http://cnn.com/2007/HEALTH/07/09/antidepressants/index.html? eref=rss_topstories

37 *half of all couples seeking therapy for marital issues have at least one clinically depressed partner:* Weeks & Gambescia, p. 178.

44 *I also bought him some L-Arginine:* L-Arginine is an amino acid, and can be purchased as a dietary supplement. There has been some preliminary evidence (but absolutely no proof) that it might be beneficial as a cure for impotence.

THREE. NOT TONIGHT, DEAR, WE'RE MARRIED

72 *Psychiatrist, sex therapist, and author Avodah Offit wrote:* Offit, Avodah K. (1981). *Night thoughts: Reflections of a sex therapist*. New York: Congdon & Lattes, p. 240.

FOUR. PREGNANCY AND THE END OF PASSION

75 *There are men who have such a strong fear of becoming a parent:* Weeks & Gambescia, p. 34.

79   *Dr. June Reinisch:* Interview with the authors July 13, 2006, and June 2, 2007. All subsequent references to Dr. Reinisch result from these interviews.

FIVE. PREDICTABLE, BORING, UNADVENTUROUS SEX

81   *it "repelled" them:* Coontz, Stephanie. (2005). *Marriage, a history.* New York: Penguin Books, p. 190.

81   *A radical Vassar college professor:* Ibid. p. 209.

81   *25 percent of American men* and *women admitted to having experienced at least one affair:* Ibid., p. 202.

82   *That belief lingered on:* Zilbergeld, Bernie. (1999). *The new male sexuality,* p. 75.

82   *Stopes warns male newlyweds:* Stopes, Marie Carmichael. (1918). *Married love: A new contribution to the solution of sex difficulties.* London: A. C. Fifield. Available online at: http://digital.library.upenn.edu/women/stopes/married/1918.html.

83   *to help alleviate hysteria:* Coontz, p. 202.

83–84   *"Every case of divorce has for its basis lack of sexual satisfaction":* Ibid., p. 204.

84   *"the multiorgasmic potential of women":* Gordon, Michael, & Shankweiler, Penelope. (August 1971). Different equals less: Female sexuality in recent marriage manuals. *Journal of Marriage and the Family,* 33, no. 3, pp. 459–466.

90   *When we asked sex therapist Janice Epp:* Online interview with the authors, July 6, 2006. All subsequent references to Dr. Epp result from this interview.

91   *"When one considers . . .":* Offit, *Night Thoughts,* p. 65.

SIX. ANGER MISMANAGEMENT

103   *a variety of ways couples deal with anger:* Weeks & Gambescia. *Hypoactive sexual desire,* pp. 61–63.

104   *Men frequently use anger to cover up sexual anxiety:* In a July 15, 2006, interview, sex therapist and educator Dr. William Stayton told the authors that some couples use fighting for the opposite reason—as aphrodisiac. These people consciously or unconsciously bait one another to stir up feelings of passion that would otherwise be dormant, like the "make-up sex" that George Costanza craves from his fiancée in an episode of *Seinfeld.* This can become an unfortunate choice: constant bickering with sex, or peace without it.

109 *Anger can also be a quiet thing:* Weeks & Gambescia. *Hypoactive sexual desire,* pp. 61–63.

109 *Dr. Robert Mendelsohn:* Interview with the authors, July 26, 2006. All subsequent references to Dr. Mendelsohn refer to this interview.

113 *Large quantities of alcohol:* Zilbergeld. *The new male sexuality,* p. 305.

SEVEN. DEPRESSION: THE ULTIMATE
PASSION KILLER

118 *The American Psychiatric Association's* Diagnostic & Statistical Manual *lists nine symptoms, which include:* DSM-IV, *Diagnostic and Statistical Manual of Mental Disorders,* Fourth Edition, American Psychiatric Association, 1994. A diagnosis of depression requires five of the symptoms within a two-week period, one of which must be a constant and pervasive feeling of depression.

119 *Some therapists claim:* Weeks & Gambescia, *Hypoactive sexual desire,* p. 50.

121 *professional help is imperative:* See the National Institute of Mental Health website for statistics and updated information about depression at www.nimh.nih.gov/publicat/depression.CFM#ptdep1. You might first want to see a family physician or specialist to rule out other factors. That physician can then refer you to a psychotherapist, psychiatrist, or psychopharmacologist.

122 *20 percent of men taking the drug experienced some dysfunction:* See www.mcmanweb.com/love_lust.htm. Refers to a 2001 study done by Dr. Anita Clayton (University of Virginia). Thirty-seven percent of the men taking antidepressants experienced sexual dysfunction. Paxil was the highest at over 40 percent; Wellbutrin the lowest at 20 percent.

124 Silk Stockings: "It's a chemical reaction, that's all." *Silk Stockings,* with music and lyrics by Cole Porter, previewed on February 24, 1955.

EIGHT. ERECTILE DYSFUNCTION: THE SILENT
PASSION KILLER

125 *Men are often ready much sooner:* On average, men can reach orgasm in four minutes, women require twenty.

126 *Multiple studies have indicated a decline in male sexual functioning after age 40:* Leiblum, Sandra R., & Segraves, R. Taylor. Sex therapy with aging adults. In Leiblum & Rosen, *Principles and practice of sex therapy,* p. 436.

126 *Lenore Tiefer interviewed hundreds of men:* Tiefer, Lenore. (1994). The medicalization of impotence. *Gender and Society, 8,* no. 3, pp. 363–377. Referenced in Bordo, p. 62.

126 *Nearly four out of ten baby boomers:* Harris Interactive survey of 1,000 men

and 1,000 women between the ages of 40 and 70, sponsored by Lily Icos LLC, the manufacturers of Cialis.

126 *websites of the big three erectile dysfunction drugs:* www.Viagra.com, www .Cialis.com, www.Levitra.com; nih/gov/1992/1992 Impotence 091/html/htm.

126 *Bob Dole and famous athletes:* Baseball star Rafael Palmeiro, was so concerned someone might actually think *he* suffered from ED that even though he endorsed Viagra in an advertising campaign, he made a hasty disclaimer to the media that he didn't really need it at all—he was just pretending.

126 *only about 20 percent of men with ED seek professional help:* Morgentaler, Abraham. (2003). *The Viagra myth.* San Francisco: Josey-Bass, an imprint of Wiley Publications, p. 12.

128 *Healthier men have an easier time getting and maintaining erections:* Esposito, K. et al. (2004). Effect of lifestyle changes on erectile dysfunction in obese men: A randomized controlled trial. *Journal of the American Medical Association, 291,* no. 24, pp. 2978–2984.

128 *shame is the primary reason men do not seek help:* Morgentaler, *The Viagra myth,* p. 13.

129 *Journalist David M. Friedman argues:* Friedman, David M. (2001). *A mind of its own.* New York, Penguin Books, pp. 304–305.

129 *Sociologists suggest:* Loe, Meika. (2004). *The rise of Viagra.* New York: New York University Press, p. 65.

130 *if a man loses his potency, he loses a part of his identity:* Friedman, *A mind of its own,* p. 304.

130 *Essayist Phillip Lopate agrees:* Lopate, Phillip. (Fall 1993). Portrait of my body. *Michigan Quarterly Review, 32,* no. 4, pp. 656–665.

130 *Sociologist Warren Farrell once mentioned:* Farrell, Warren. (1986). *Why men are the way they are.* New York: Berkley, p. 265.

130 *allowing Tom Wolfe to wittily call impotence:* Wolfe, Tom. (2000). *Hooking up.* New York: Picador, p. 9.

130 *A 1990 study found:* Weeks & Gambescia, *Hypoactive sexual desire,* p. 44.

131 *If the problem is physical:* Morgentaler, *The Viagra myth,* p. 12.

133 *For men with psychological impotence:* Ibid.

133 *this decreases to about 65 percent:* Ibid., pp. 142–143.

134 *If the drugs prove ineffective, there are other paths to explore:* Friedman, *A mind of its own,* p. 302, quoting urologist and impotency specialist Dr. Gregory Broderick.

134 *Sociologist Susan Bordo recommends:* Bordo, Susan. (1999). *The male body.* New York: Farrar, Straus and Giroux, pp. 64–65.

135 *Abraham Morgentaler elegantly suggests:* Morgentaler, *The Viagra myth,* p. 65.

141 *The American Psychiatric Association defines rapid ejaculation as follows:* DSM-IV, American Psychiatric Association, 1994, 302.75.

141 *Rapid ejaculation has more recently been defined:* http://www.cumc.columbia

.edu/dept/urology/ErectileDysfunction_prem.html; also see Polonsky, Derek C. Premature ejaculation. In Leiblum & Rosen, pp. 305–332.

141   *Twenty-five percent of American men:* National Health and Social life Survey (NHSLS), 1992.

142   *The fallacy with this approach:* See Schnarch, *Resurrecting sex,* pp. 259–265.

143   *it has been theorized that certain men are so anxious to please:* Apfelbaum, Bernard. "Retarded ejaculation: A much misunderstood syndrome." In Leiblum & Rosen, pp. 205–241.

NINE. CAUGHT IN THE NET

145   *When Shere Hite compiled her two classic statistical volumes:* Hite, Shere. (1976). *The Hite report: A nationwide study on female sexuality.* New York: Macmillan, p. 13.

145   *"almost all men, whether married or single":* Hite, Shere. (1981). *The Hite report on male sexuality.* New York: Alfred A. Knopf, p. 485.

146   *"Whether we share our sexuality becomes a matter of choice, not obligation":* Offit, *Night thoughts,* p. 174.

146   *the musical* Avenue Q: Lopez, Robert, & Marx, Jeff. *Avenue Q* opened July 31, 2003. The title of the song referred to is: "The Internet Is for Porn."

146   *an estimated $10 billion industry:* Loe, *The rise of Viagra,* p. 65.

146   *"Porn is as old as the cave painting":* Dr. Joy Browne, interview with the authors, July 17, 2006.

148   *Swiss psychiatrist Auguste Henri-Forel warned:* Stopes, *Married love,* chapter 3.

148   *"marriages are briefer than at any time since this nation began":* Hacker, Andrew. (2003). *Mismatch: The growing gulf between men and women.* New York: Scribner, p. 13.

149   *Internet pornography has little in common with the kind of sex we really experience:* Ken Search, LCSW, interview with the authors, July 3, 2006.

149   *a digital divide like the one Tom Wolfe mentions:* Wolfe, *Hooking up,* p. 9.

152   *Dr. Julian Slowinski:* Interview with the authors, July 14, 2006. All subsequent references to Dr. Slowinski result from this interview.

152   *'you are as guilty for the thought as you are for the deed':* Dr. Fitzgerald's biblical quotation is a variation of Matt. 5:21–28: "If you have ever thought a lustful thought you are guilty of adultery."

153   *When Bob wrote* His Secret Life: Berkowitz, Bob. (1997). *His secret life.* New York: Simon & Schuster.

153   *Fantasies do change over time:* Weeks & Gambescia, *Hypoactive sexual desire,* p. 27.

153–54 *Some consider Internet addiction to be growing so rapidly they regard it as an epidemic:* Ibid., pp. 48–49.

154 *"most worrisome" about online pornography:* Leiblum & Rosen, *Principles and practice of sex therapy,* p. 10.

154 *The* New York Times *reports:* Kershaw, Sarah. Hooked on the web: Help is on the way. *New York Times.* December 1, 2005.

154 *Otherwise the patient would pay out of pocket:* Kershaw.

154–55 *pornography addicts suffer from a combination of emotional immaturity, lack of discipline, and a fear of intimacy:* Jay Parker, interview with the authors, June 30, 2006.

TEN. NO SEX PLEASE, WE'RE EATING

163 *"lack of attraction to partner, usually weight gain" can be a primary causative:* LoPiccolo, Joseph, & Friedman, Jerry. (1988). Broad spectrum treatment of low sexual desire: Integration of cognitive, behavioral, and systemic therapy. In Leiblum, S. R., & Rosen, R. C. (Eds.), *Sexual Desire Disorders* (pp. 125–126). New York: Guilford Press.

164 *A recent Tufts University School of Medicine study:* Anderson, Sarah, & Must, Aviva. *Pediatrics and adolescent medicine,* March 2006.

165 *Hilde Bruch:* Bruch, Hilde. (1997). Body image and self-awareness. In Counihan, Carole, & Van Esterik, Penny (Eds.), *Food and culture.* New York: Routledge, pp. 218–220.

167 *a national survey on women, weight, sex, and marriage:* Stuart, Richard B., & Jacobson, Barbara. (1987). *Weight, sex, and marriage.* New York: W.W. Norton & Company.

168 *"The emphasis on appearance [can be] a red herring":* Weeks & Gambescia, p. 41.

169 *an example of a man falsely blaming impotence on his wife's obesity:* Stuart & Jacobson, *Weight, sex, and marriage,* p. 51.

ELEVEN. MAYBE HE'S GAY? ASEXUAL?

176 *The University of Chicago's seminal 1994 survey:* Michael, Robert T., Gagnon, John H., Laumann, Edward O., & Kolata, Gina. (1999). *Sex in America: A definitive survey.* Boston: Little, Brown and Company, pp. 174–176.

176 *"3.9 percent of American men who had ever been married had sex with men in the previous five years":* Butler, Katy. Many couples must negotiate terms of brokeback marriages. *New York Times,* March 7, 2006.

176 *Support for same-sex marriage has been tabulated as high as 40 percent:* Coontz, *Marriage: A history,* p. 274.

176 *in America's twelve largest cities the gay population is estimated to be, on average, 9 percent:* Michael et al. *Sex in America,* p. 177.

177   *"These individuals may not wish to admit to themselves they are gay"*: Weeks & Gambescia, p. 47.

177   *"brokeback marriages"*: Butler, *New York Times,* March 7, 2006. We first came across the term "brokeback marriage" in this article.

182   *There is a broad range of possible levels of sexual desire:* Baumeister, R. F., Catanese, K. R., & Vohs, K. D. (2001). Is there a gender difference in strength of sex drives? Theoretical views, conceptual distinctions, and a review of relevant evidence. *Personality and Social Psychology Review, 5,* no. 3, pp. 242–273.

183   *In a 1991 study:* Ibid., p. 243.

183   *A 1995 study concluded:* Ibid.

183   *A 2001 extensive review:* Ibid.

183   *in a 2006 online survey:* www.msnbc.msn.com/id/12410076.

183   *The American Psychiatric Association defines it like this:* American Psychiatric Association. (2000). *Diagnostic and statistical manual of mental disorders* (4th ed., DSM-IV).

184   *Studies have shown it to be more prevalent in females:* Weeks & Gambescia, *Hypoactive sexual desire,* p. ix, in reference to an analysis of the United States National Health and Social Life Survey (Laumann, Paik, Rosen, 1999).

184   *the statistics regarding frequency of intercourse for married couples:* Ibid., p. 29.

184   *Therapist Michele Weiner Davis states:* Davis, Michele Weiner. (2003). *The sex-starved marriage.* New York: Simon & Schuster, p. 25.

186   *Asexuals Have Other Things on Their Minds:* This saying is printed on a T-shirt available at the AVEN online retail store. www.asexuality.org.

186   *researcher Anthony Bogaert published a national study:* Bogaert, Anthony. (2004). Asexuality: Prevalence and associated factors in a national probability sample. *Journal of Sex Research, 41,* no. 3, pp. 279–287.

188   *The Massachusetts Male Aging study assessed the sex drive:* Travison, T. G., Morley, J. E., Araujo, A. B., O'Donnell, A. B., & McKinlay, J. B. (July 2006). The Relationship between libido and testosterone levels in aging men. In *Journal of Clinical Endocrinology and Metabolism,* 91, no. 7, pp. 2509–2513.

189   *In animal testing, males deprived of testosterone:* Morgentaler, Abraham. (1993). *The male body.* New York: Simon & Schuster, p. 133.

189   *The Massachusetts Male Aging Study estimated that there were about 2.4 million 40- to 69-year-old men in America with a testosterone deficiency:* Andre, B., Araujo, A. B., O'Donnell, A. B., Brambilla, D. J., Simpson, W. B., Longcope, C., Matsumoto, A. M., & McKinlay, J. B. (December 2004). Prevalence and incidence of androgen deficiency in middle-aged and older men: Estimates from the Massachusetts Male Aging Study. In *Journal of Clinical Endocrinology & Metabolism,* 89, no. 12, pp. 5920–5926.

189   *the "so-called syndrome called andropause"*: Friedman, Richard A. The waist may expand, but the libido stays fit. *New York Times,* October 24, 2006.

TWELVE. SHOULD I STAY OR SHOULD I GO?

195   *Half of all marriages in America end*: Hacker, *Mismatch*, p. 198. The National Center for Health Statistics, 2001, forecast that first marriages of persons then aged 25 stood a 52.5 percent chance of ending in divorce. Statistics vary by age and other demographics. See http://www.cdc.gov/nchs/.

197   *According to sociologist Paul Amato*: Coontz, *Marriage: A history,* p. 293.

THIRTEEN. WHAT WOMEN ARE DOING ABOUT IT

206   *'Men who have a low drive for sex have an even lower drive for sex therapy'*: Dr. Joseph LoPiccolo, part of response to authors' question, via e-mail, October 24, 2006.

208   *You can get referrals from . . . the APA website*: See www.apa.org. Click on "Find a psychologist."

209   *How long should therapy last?* Carey, Benedict. An analyst questions the self-perpetuating side of therapy. *New York Times,* October 10, 2006.

FOURTEEN. AND IN THE END . . .

210   *the love you take is equal to the love you make?*: Lennon, John, & McCartney, Paul. "The End," *Abbey Road*, released September 26, 1969.

acknowledgments

Many people contributed to this project, but none with greater impact than our thousands of survey respondents. We are aware of how difficult it is to even anonymously discuss intimate and sometimes painful issues; these people responded with courage, bravery, and eloquence.

The book would have never been written without the enthusiasm of Peter Hubbard, our extraordinary editor at HarperCollins/Morrow. He believed in this topic and its importance right from the start, and his insightful suggestions and editorial comments were always on track. We are grateful as well to our excellent copyeditor, Laurie McGee.

Sharon Whiteley, Melissa Gleason, and Karin Bilich of the wonderful website ThirdAge.com were invaluable in their professionalism and support—the majority of our survey participants reached us through their online magazine.

Our thanks as well to our friend Dr. Stephen Gessner, who was kind enough to read our manuscript and give so many smart suggestions, most of which we immediately incorporated into the text.

Many people generously shared their wisdom and time: Linda Ballew, Dr. Bernard Berkowitz, Dr. Joy Browne, Dr. Janice Epp, Dr. Helen Fisher, Dr. Della Fitzgerald, Dr. Max Fitzgerald, Dr. Thomas

A. Foster, Dr. Joseph LoPiccolo, Dr. Bob Mendelsohn, Jay Parker, Dr. June Reinisch, Ken Search, Dr. Julian Slowinski, Dr. William Stayton, and Liana Zhou. We are deeply grateful to you all.

Thanks as well to Dr. David Hall for his assistance in setting up our survey, to our friend Bill Bernstein, and to Roger Yager for all of their help and support.

Lastly, we thank all of our friends and family who were sympathetic with our lack of availability—indeed, cloistered existence—during the long periods researching and writing this book, when our only companions were the always interesting and amusing cats, Freddie and D. J., and each other, which, incidentally, worked out far better than we had even dared to dream.

index